When Hope Overcame the Impossible

An epic story of a thirteen-year-old boy who
refused the death sentence of brain cancer!

Thomas M Walsh
Sept. 3, 2021

Thomas M. Walsh

www.TotalPublishingAndMedia.com

ISBN 978-1-63302-177-8

What People Are Saying About the Author and This Book:

Tom Walsh and his wife are dedicated and compassionate educators in our community. When their world flipped upside down, Sapulpa and many others around the State of Oklahoma and Tennessee pulled together for them. Prayers were lifted for the family and Isaac as they entered this journey in battling cancer. Our lives were touched, in many ways changed, by their steadfast belief God has a plan for this family and Isaac. A great read for anyone that is on the 'roller coaster' ride of dealing with their child in a fight for their life.

Claudia Bartlett
Oklahoma Foundation for Excellence in Public Education
Oklahoma State University Foundation Board of Governors

Tom Walsh was always considered a caring top notch educator, and a principal who could turn around a school in need of leadership. It wasn't until the wrenching medical journey of his son, Isaac, that the entire community understood the faith and perseverance Tom and his family possessed. Tom's heartfelt story shares the family's constant trust in God and love for their son.

Dr. Mary Webb
Superintendent of Sapulpa Public Schools (Retired)
Sapulpa, Oklahoma

Tom has given us an image of what pediatric cancer looks like through the eyes of a parent. There could be no better advocate for parents in their journey through childhood cancer. God has truly held the hands of the Walsh family.

Jennifer Holt
Third Grade Teacher, Liberty Elementary STEM Academy
Sapulpa, Oklahoma

From the beginning Tom and Dacia Walsh put "normal life" on hold to support their son Isaac, in the wake of the diagnosis of his pediatric brain tumor. Like so many St. Jude families they made deep personal sacrifices to put "first things first" in a time of crisis. For this family that meant prioritizing their time together as a family, learning more about medical issues than they ever wanted to know, and constantly showering their son with a love that would sustain him through a terribly difficult time. They were held together by wonderful family relationships, and by a faith that enabled them to recognize God's blessing were available to them both in times of fear and of joy. Whether the news was hopeful or frightening, this family was secure in their trust that nothing in all creation could separate them from God's love. It was a remarkable thing to be part of, and I'm most grateful for the privilege of having been there to be part of it.

Mark Brown, MDiv, BCC
Spiritual Care Services
St. Jude Children's Research Hospital
Memphis, Tennessee

Getting to hear Tom Walsh's perspective, and learning of his son's cancer fight and the way St. Jude touched his family, really opens your eyes to the struggles families face, and puts our smaller worries into perspective. As many families have told me, when your child becomes a St. Jude patient, you become a member of an exclusive 'club' that you never wanted to join. Even when your child completes treatment, you are part of the St. Jude family for the rest of your life. Tom is so authentic when he shares his family's experience. You will love reading Isaac's story, and cheering him on, against the odds.

Michelle Linn
Morning News Anchor and Investigative Reporter
Tulsa's Fox 23 News (CMG – TV)
Tulsa, Oklahoma

Tom Walsh is an extraordinary family man, leader, and educator. Over the years he has guided children through the challenging rites of passage, encompassing elementary and middle school. In addition, he has developed and mentored educational strategies which will lead children to become integral members of society. Tom has shown his unwavering faith when tested beyond parental limits with his older son's battle with pediatric brain cancer. His dedication to bring attention and support to others who face tragedies is a testament to his remarkable character, and commitment to improving children's' lives.

Stefanie Gilbert
5th grade Teacher, Liberty Elementary STEM Academy
Sapulpa, Oklahoma

Tom's life as a principal showed not only care and compassion, he was also an inspiration to each of his students. When Isaac was diagnosed with cancer, the same care and compassion spilled over into the lives of everyone they came in contact with throughout their journey. He gave unselfishly of himself to assure not only Isaac, but others that faith in God would see them through. A strong faith and inspiration have led him to write this book - to share just how powerful our God is.

Dr. Richard and Mrs. Janet Pitts
Godparents to Isaac and Caleb Walsh
Sapulpa, Oklahoma

I have the privilege of working with Tom Walsh over the past five years. I can say his life is an inspiration to all! Although he and his family have faced many challenges, his optimism combined with faith and a drive to overcome barriers has never failed. His journey provided guidance and encouragement for all.

Kimberly Collier
President
Collier Consulting LLC
Edmond, Oklahoma

While Tom's contributions to his community and church are many, the impact of their experience as they walked through this season were profound on all those who knew them. We are grateful to call Tom and his family lifelong friends and encourage you to read the story of a family's faith, young boy's courage, and a great God.

Lynnette Kautz
Advanced Director with the Pampered Chef
Kellyville, Oklahoma

When life gives you hurdles, it is best to jump over them with grace. This is what Tom Walsh has shown everyone that knows him. I am so grateful to not only call him my mentor and former colleague, but my friend. He has used Isaac's story to inspire, console, and educate those who may be experiencing a very difficult time in their lives. I hope as you read his story, you feel the passion and love he has for his family.

Bridget Hailey
Principal, Jefferson Heights Elementary
Sapulpa, Oklahoma

Traveling the journey of childhood cancer takes resiliency, grit, and unwavering hope, all of which Tom Walsh tirelessly showed day after day, and month after month in the fight for his son's life. His desire for his son Isaac to be healed is a resounding feeling that parents can relate to, no matter their circumstances. Tom writes to show his son's path to health but gives so much more in faith and unwavering determination to always do what is best for your child.

Rebecca Clostio
Third Grade Teacher, Jefferson Heights Elementary
Sapulpa, Oklahoma

I've known Tom for more than twenty-five years. We first met when Tom was a Spanish teacher at Sapulpa Junior High, and I was the assistant principal. I became close to Isaac and Caleb over the years. They were both really good athletes and I often attended their elementary basketball and soccer games. Isaac was left-handed and had a great arm. I once remarked that Isaac's left arm may be the key to Tom's early retirement one day. I saw Major League Baseball in Isaac's future. However, in 2011 those dreams were jeopardized. I had season tickets to the

University of Tulsa. Tom and his boys would regularly go with me to the games. Isaac was the most passionate of all of us and I could always count on him going to a game even if Tom and Caleb could not go. In the spring of 2011, we were at a game and Isaac got dizzy. He wanted to go home which I found very strange. He also wasn't hungry which was very unusual for Isaac. A few days later, Tom called to tell me Isaac had been diagnosed with brain cancer. Isaac's story, as told by his father will inspire you in a way only a child who faced death three times and never gave up hope can do.

Jim Baird
Family friend and retired school administrator
Tulsa, Oklahoma

Tom Walsh has been a friend to his community throughout his entire career as an educator and administrator. Nothing speaks more of his character than how his peers and his community treated his family during this time of trial. The community raised money for his travel expenses and fellow educators donated their vacation time so Tom and Dacia could spend time with Isaac without missing a paycheck.

James "Rusty" Kautz
First United Bank Investment Broker
Sapulpa, Oklahoma

Dedicated to the Children of St. Jude

Your courage inspires us.
The attitude in which you face adversity comforts our souls.
May peace and hope forever fill your hearts with joy.
You had cancer but cancer never had you!

For Isaac and Caleb

True Heroes and Warriors
Your Lives are an Inspiration to Us All

Table of Contents

Reverend Mark Brown, MDiv, BCC Spiritual Care Services, St. Jude Children's Research Hospital in Memphis, TN

Dr. Mary Webb *(Retired)* Superintendent of Sapulpa Public Schools

Jennifer Poyner, Sr. Advisor of Special Projects and Integration at St. Jude Children's Research Hospital in Memphis, TN

Juana McCoy, Former owner of Zoe Memphis Boutique in Memphis, TN

James Womack, Former Head Coach of the Sapulpa High School Chieftains Boys Basketball Team

Nate Tibbetts, Associate Head Coach of the NBA Portland Trail Blazers

The NBA Cares

Meri Armour, President *(Retired)* of Le Bonheur Children's Hospital in Memphis, TN

Joan Eisenstodt, Owner of Eisenstodt Associates LLC in Washington DC

Jon Greer, Sapulpa First Church of God Youth Pastor

Michelle Linn, Morning Anchor and Photojournalist at Tulsa's Fox 23 News

Dr. Richard and Mrs. Janet Pitts, Godparents of Isaac and Caleb Walsh

Earl and Sandy Blevins, Oklahoma Make a Wish
  Foundation

Nicole Doyle, Senior Season Ticket Account Manager for
  the NBA Oklahoma City Thunder

Brian Davis, Fox Sports TV Play by Play Voice *(Retired)*
  of the NBA Oklahoma City Thunder

Acknowledgements

I'm often asked why it took nine years after Isaac's cancer diagnosis to write his story. In some ways I believe the uncertainty of Isaac's recovery hardened in me a yearning to see how his life evolved. More so, it was when I made the decision to retire from public education in January 2020, did my desire to spread an awareness of pediatric cancer become the driving force to write this book.

Mark Twain is considered by many to be one of the greatest American authors of all time. I think he said it best when he wrote…

"Writing is easy.
All you have to do is cross out the wrong words."

I'm thankful for the encouragement of Suzanne Shirey *(President, Sapulpa Area Chamber of Commerce)* for suggesting I write Isaac's story. It was also through Suzanne I came into contact with the editorial team of Total Publishing and Media LLC. They in essence helped me *"Cross out the wrong words,"* and make my first attempt at professional writing come to fruition.

No book is ever possible without the devotion of friends and family who provide encouraging words when the easier route is to give up on a laborious task. I'm appreciative of three of my former staff members: Rebecca Clostio, Jennifer Holt and Luanne Guerrero for reading my numerous drafts and providing me with timely feedback. Your comments and opinions gave me the courage to finish my final draft. Notwithstanding, my youngest brother Jon is a self-published author himself. He gave me the inspiration to follow in his footsteps.

No finished work is ever complete without the blessing of your spouse. I'm thankful for my wife Dacia. Her steadfast devotion and support gave me the desire to see this to the end.

My aspiration is the pages which follow will bring hope to the brokenhearted and healing to the emotionally bruised. I often tell people no one is ever cured of cancer. Rather, they survive and learn to live life with the handicaps and disabilities their treatment has left behind. As for me, I will never be the same as a result of watching my young son battle cancer. He is my hero and serves as a motivation to be a part of the search for a cure to this dreadful disease.

Preface

E ach year approximately three-hundred-fifty children are diagnosed with medulloblastoma *(muh-dul-o-blas-toe-muh)* brain cancer in the United States. Comprising nearly twenty percent of all malignant brain tumors diagnosed, medulloblastomas are the most common form of brain cancer in children. According to St. Jude, most medulloblastoma tumors occur in children under the age of sixteen. Further, the disease is more common in boys than girls. Lastly, although rare, some young adults in their 20's have been diagnosed with a medulloblastoma brain tumor. The cause of medulloblastomas is unknown. However, research has determined children are born with the fetal cancerous cells stored in their brain.

Medulloblastomas often form in the back lower part of the brain known as the cerebellum. This area of the brain controls fine motor skills, balance and movement. Due to the tumor's location within the central nervous system, they often spread down the spinal cord and may form in clusters of more than one.

Treatment for a medulloblastoma generally involves surgery to resect *(remove)* the tumor combined with radiation and chemotherapy to kill off any remaining cancerous cells in the spinal fluid. St. Jude has made tremendous discoveries regarding the molecular makeup of the medulloblastoma tumor and now classifies them as four types. Depending upon the classification, the amount of radiation and chemotherapy is adjusted.

The survival rate at St. Jude for a medulloblastoma is from seventy to eighty percent. However, if the tumor has spread down the spinal cord the rate is lower; by this time more than one tumor has likely been detected. Survival rates for tumors which have spread down the spine are roughly sixty percent.

The pages which follow detail my son Isaac's epic battle against medulloblastoma brain cancer. Isaac was thirteen years old at the time of his diagnosis. His worst medical problem prior to cancer was an ear infection. As with most families who care for a cancer-stricken child, there is no book, YouTube video, nor step-sheet on how to prepare for such a catastrophe. Rather, we learn from those wounded warriors who have fought the battle before our own. More so, for every family it's a fight to overcome the societal attitude which decries cancer as a sentence of death. It's often been said the hopes and dreams of tomorrow reside in the hearts of children. Maybe one day the need for a St. Jude will be no more. When this does happen, I am certain there will be smiles from those who have given their life's work to see this dream come true.

Foreword

T om Walsh describes in the upcoming book the journey of his son through a complex cancer diagnosis and treatment. The story of Isaac is one of courage and resilience. Further, of a boy turned young man who found the grit and tenacity to see his way to the other side of cancer. Isaac is a remarkable example of "one day at a time." His story and that of his parents who journeyed with him side by side, is a rollercoaster ride of ups and downs. Isaac and his family are examples of quiet determination and mutual support.

Tom Wash writes from the perspective of a life-long educator. He observes, analyzes and offers his observations of our healthcare system as it whirled around Isaac and family. Tom's vantage point is unique in how he chooses to see the better angels in a healthcare system which sometimes succeeded and occasionally failed in Isaac's care. However, this story is one of a true partnership between Isaac, his parents and caregivers. The story is filled with examples of kindness, concern and learning by a team of healthcare professionals who treated Isaac.

During Isaac's illness and rehabilitation, he was a patient at Le Bonheur Children's Hospital in Memphis, Tennessee. Le Bonheur is a partner hospital to St. Jude Children's Research Hospital. I was the CEO at Le Bonheur (2007-2019) during the time Isaac was a patient with us. I am also a nurse by background and my areas of experience were oncology and pediatrics. I met Isaac and family on one of his first admissions to Le Bonheur. At the time, I did not realize the impact Isaac's story would have on me and on the staff of Le Bonheur. After a failed reanimation graft, Tom Walsh and I met to talk about how to improve for the next attempt. Tom was insightful and recognized the incredible responsibility and commitment the staff had for Isaac's best care. Tom told me about the PICU nurses who called or came in on their days off to check on Isaac. Notwithstanding, describing the tremendous show of compassion by the plastic surgeon who spent the night by Isaac's bedside. Tom found strength in their commitment and kindness. One should never forget the impact every caregiver has on a patient and their family. We worked hard as a team of surgeons, nurses and hospital administration with Tom to make Isaac's second reanimation graft attempt successful. The impact Isaac had on Le Bonheur was that of a change agent. We got better because of Tom's engagement and Isaac's courage.

As you read this story of Isaac, I hope it brings you a new understanding of how resilience manifests itself in the most difficult of situations, of how parents endure and support a child even when their hearts are filled with trepidation. Additionally, how a healthcare team can love and care for a child and their family. Lastly, of how a team can always improve in their partnership with families.

Isaac is a brave young man now onto the next chapters in his life. You will in reading his story, through the eyes of his father, be undoubtedly left believing there is always hope and "the better angels," surround you during tough times. It is a beautiful story and one only a loving father could write.

Meri Armour, MSN, MBA
Retired President & CEO
Le Bonheur Children's Hospital
Memphis, TN

Part I
Early Diagnosis

Painful Memories

Concordia, Kansas
July 25, 2012

I t was a hot and humid mid-summer day in this rural farming community in north central Kansas. Known for its hometown friendly atmosphere and wheat production, this was the place where I grew up as a child. I had returned many times to see my sister who was the only one in our family of eight kids who settled in Concordia. My visit however, would be more than just seeing family. I had come to reminisce about my childhood and contemplate what my family's future would hold.

I parked my car near the long-abandoned McKinley Elementary School where my younger brothers had attended class. The playground which once was home to the laughter and play of children was marked now by large cracks in the asphalt with overgrown weeds. As I walked across the school yard, I was drawn to where an eight-foot basketball goal was once tucked by the side of the building. I remember the day this goal was installed brand new. The backboard was white and the curved pole a shiny silver. As a young child, I would spend hours playing in this spot. Like many school age children I idolized sports celebrities. It was my dream to play in the National Basketball Association (NBA), and in many ways my childhood dreams became a reality in the world of my playful imagination; on this outdoor basketball court I was a professional athlete.

Today the abandoned elementary school and forgotten basketball goal mirrored my somber mood. My 14 year old son Isaac had just completed a ten-month treatment protocol for pediatric brain cancer, *(Medulloblastoma - PNET; stage III & grade IV)* at St. Jude Children's Research Hospital in Memphis, Tennessee. The experimental therapy had left him emotionally bruised, physically scarred and fighting lifelong disabilities. Tears filled my eyes as I contemplated what his childhood dreams would be. Did this dreadful disease rob him of the innocence of childhood? What would his hopes and desires be for his future? Most importantly, what would the future hold for him and our family?

This book is more than just a father's account of his child's battle with cancer. It's about an entire community which rallied around a family to save a young life in crisis. The following pages reveal a team of dedicated medical professionals at St. Jude Children's Research Hospital whose sole mission is finding a cure to save children from this horrible illness. Lastly, if not for the painstakingly hard work of the army of fundraising agents who comprise ALSAC, the fundraising and awareness organization of the hospital, children like Isaac would never have a chance to fulfill their dreams. *When Hope Overcame the Impossible* is where cancer meets its most fierce opponent, the hearts of those who refuse to be broken by this devastating disease.

One Gold Coin

M y wife Dacia and I were married in Tulsa, Oklahoma on May 7, 1989. After settling into careers as educators in a neighboring school district called Sapulpa Public Schools, our desire was to start a family, a desire wrought with difficulties. Taking the path many weary couples take, our inability to conceive a child led us to seek medical intervention with a fertility specialist.

In the early 1990's fertility treatment was in its infancy. The procedure would not be covered by our insurance and the success rate was less than twenty-five percent. The doctor explained the fertility treatments would require Dacia to make daily trips to his office. She would undergo numerous injections to create a human egg. In all, the treatments would cost in excess of twenty-five thousand dollars and there was no guarantee it would produce a human embryo.

After a series of tests, Dacia and I went to meet with the doctor to hear his proposed treatment plan. His words echoed like the sound of a glass vase breaking on a ceramic floor. "You have no chance of conceiving a child unless you seek fertility treatments." I sat in stunned silence as I pondered life without the sound of children in our home. Dacia found the thought of motherhood passing her over, and the realization adoption would be our only path to have children deeply disappointing. However, she would not let the doctor's diagnosis become an avenue to blame her. As for me, struggling to form my words, I asked the young doctor, "You mean to tell me without medical intervention, we will never be able to start a family on our own?"

He answered my question with an analogy. "Say you were to fill the entire state of Texas with silver dollars a foot deep and hid one gold coin among them, then tried to find the gold coin with a swipe of the hand, that's how much chance you have of conceiving a child."

We found that gold coin nearly four years later to the day when Isaac Daniel Walsh was born on July 21, 1997. He was a healthy child brought into this world without fertility treatments. Two years later, Dacia gave birth to our second child Caleb Thomas Walsh who also was born without the intervention of a medical procedure.

Isaac's birth in some respects symbolized something special for me. He was the son I was told we could never conceive on our own and a child of promise. Years prior, I had come to the realization my heart would be left to find solace in loving someone else's child. His childhood represented through life's most bitter disappointments, there is hope for those who refuse to be defined by the impossible.

Little did I know thirteen years later, tragedy would strike our family. Cancer had shown up on our doorstep and marked our first born. Thrown into a hurried state of making life and death decisions, and staring over an abyss contemplating the loss of my oldest son, this calamity would leave me questioning my faith.

Warning Signs

The sound of the crowd cheering filled the basketball gymnasium at Sapulpa Junior High School. A thirteen-year-old redheaded seventh grader had just entered the game. He was known as the team's sixth man and their clutch three-point shooter. His lanky legs were reminiscent of a typical teenager whose coordination was trying to catch up with the adolescent changes going on in his body. Tonight he was lethargic and listless. Sprinting onto the floor, he knew something was wrong. Usually overjoyed at his chance to play, he reluctantly signaled the coach and asked to be pulled from the court. Complaining of a headache, short of breath and legs hurting; Isaac Walsh had just played his last basketball game.

In some respects, this fateful contest was a turning point in Isaac's young life. Driving home from the game in the darkness of night, Isaac complained his vision was blurry and he could not read the signs by the side of the road. Initially, I attributed his intermittent poor vision to a winter fog which hung in the valleys, and at times made driving difficult in the rolling hills of Sapulpa. Days later a phone call from the school informing us Isaac had fainted in the hallway sent us to our family physician searching for answers.

The weeks which followed were filled with numerous visits to medical specialists. A vision exam cleared Isaac of any eye disease, a trip to the chiropractor ruled out a herniated disc, lab results from the doctor's office were negative for rheumatoid arthritis and a trip to the emergency room diagnosed him as a little dehydrated. Despite all the seemingly good news from the medical tests, Isaac's condition was deteriorating by the day.

I clearly remember the last day I dropped him off at school before he was admitted to the hospital. As Isaac walked gingerly across the cement schoolyard, he positioned his head in an awkward manner as if to relieve some type of pressure in his neck. Isaac had lost thirty pounds or nearly twenty-five percent of his body weight. Due to the lack of food intake and the toll this illness was taking on his body, he appeared ghostly white in color. His ghastly appearance attracted a group of student onlookers who stared at him as if he were from another planet. My hands began to shake as I gripped the steering wheel of the car. A deep sadness came over me as I watched my child being undeservingly thrust into a world of childhood ridicule. The anguish and pain I felt left me feeling powerless, as my search for answers had yielded nothing.

Deeply alarmed and concerned, I called our doctor and pleaded for something to end this nightmare. I vividly remember what she told me, "Do not go anywhere, I'm going to call and get some tests ordered." Roughly one hour later, on March 8, 2011 Isaac was admitted to St. Francis Children's Hospital in Tulsa, Oklahoma. The doctor had ordered a CT scan of his brain and spine. We were told a few hours later the scan showed an "abnormality" and a doctor would come and talk to us soon. His room was quiet and void of activity throughout the night. Reluctantly, I drifted off into fitful and disturbed sleep as I pondered what exactly the scan had revealed. I awoke a few hours later to the sound of a large wooden door opening from the hall into our room. A young female doctor appeared and in a very calm professional manner asked if we had any questions about the results of the scan.

"You really don't know"

The doctor's reassuring demeanor gave me the sense of peace I had been ardently wanting from the results of the many tests which had been done. I told the doctor we knew the CT scan showed an abnormality, and details would be discussed with us later. In a brief second her disposition changed. Her stunned and perplexed facial expression sent chills down my spine. An overarching sensation of fear overwhelmed me. Gathering her thoughts, she said, "You really don't know, do you?"

Knowing what she had to say next would be upsetting, she asked us to follow her to a consult room. Carefully choosing her words, and in a somber voice, I remember her saying, "The scan has revealed Isaac has a brain tumor. We believe due to its location on the brain stem, it's malignant and a form of cancer."

Nothing in life had prepared me for this day. In an instant I found myself at a total loss for words - unable to comprehend the impact on our lives this diagnosis would bring. Cancer had taken the life of my mother-in-law, my mother and now indiscriminately laid claim to my first-born son. Dacia, overcome with grief, recalled struggling to speak due to difficulty breathing. We realized we had to get back to Isaac's room. Wiping tears from my eyes and struggling to find the words to utter we embraced. I asked Dacia, "What do we tell Isaac, what do we say to our son?"

Saying Goodbye

We arrived back at the room only to be met with a flurry of questions from Isaac. We told him very little, as there was no clear diagnosis or plan to move forward. However, Isaac perceived something was wrong. He asked us to hold his hand as he was afraid of what might happen next. I watched signs of anxiety build to a climax when he asked if he was going to die. In my brokenness and sorrow, I could only answer I didn't know as more tests had to be done. However, like Isaac, I too was afraid this could be the end.

Shortly after arriving in his room a knock on the door alerted me to a neurosurgeon standing in the hall. He asked me to step into a consultation area so we could discuss Isaac's condition. He showed me the CT scan taken shortly after Isaac was admitted to the hospital. The scan confirmed my worst fears, Isaac clearly had a tumor in his brain. It was the surgeon's opinion that it was malignant. He said the pathology lab would determine the type of cancer and what further treatment would entail.

The surgeon's words rang hollow as if I were in a dream. He told me Isaac would require immediate surgery. The hours long operation involved drilling a reservoir hole through the skull into his brain to alleviate the pressure the tumor was causing - the tumor could not be removed until the pressure could be equalized. This was an extremely risky and dangerous procedure. He told me to prepare for Isaac's passing, as it was expected he would die of a stroke and/or heart attack on the operating table. With my hand shaking, and visibly distraught, I took the pen from the doctor and signed the surgery consent forms. "Mr. Walsh, in signing this consent form you must understand this is a dangerous operation, there is an extremely high-risk Isaac will die today." These words are etched in my memory as if penned on a gravestone.

Isaac's vital signs were erratic. The tumor had cut off spinal fluid and blood to his brain. The onset of seizures caused unconsciousness. Lying in a hospital bed in a fetal position, Isaac's body movements were slow and lifeless. In my state of anguish and pain, I discerned the end of Isaac's young life about to unfold before me. I was overcome with grief when a team of nurses showed up at the door to take him off to surgery. Trembling and finding my words difficult to form, I whispered in his ear, "I love you son. I'll see you again in paradise."

As the large metal doors to the surgery area closed, I realized my family would be different now. Isaac's life would either end in a funeral or miraculously a fierce battle would ensue to eradicate cancer from his feeble body. A few moments later we were directed to the surgery waiting area. A nurse said the team would call us with updates throughout the three-hour operation. Sitting on a hard-padded chair listening for the phone to ring, I began to reminisce about a young boy caught between the clutches of life, and perils of death.

Forty-Five Minutes of Silence

The waiting room was nearly empty as most surgeries had been completed by the midday hour. The operation had come so suddenly only a few family members and close friends were in the lobby awaiting word from the surgical team. There was a lonely eerie silence among all who had gathered. Despite being able to accept losing my mother to cancer two years prior, I found no hope of being able to heal after losing a child.

Anticipating the phone might ring any minute, I began to prepare for what appeared to be the impending passing of my son. I found my thoughts suspended, as if in the midst of a dream, hoping when I awoke it would all be over. Reflecting on Isaac's childhood brought a deep sense of sorrow as I began to contemplate life's traditions without him. I found a distracted calmness focusing on the rays of sun flooding the room. Fixated on the sunlight stretching across the room to my feet, I noticed a shadow under the base of the door. Puzzled and somewhat concerned, I heard movement in the hallway. From the corner of my eye I saw a man wearing surgical gear enter the waiting room. Coming to brief us only forty-five minutes after surgery began was our surgeon, I arose to greet him but found I was unable to speak. Isaac might have died at the start of the operation. Death must have come early in the surgery. Yet, the surgeon's demeanor did not indicate what he had to say was unpleasant. Rather, he smiled before he spoke.

He told us Isaac was alive and did not suffer a stroke during surgery. Further, he said Isaac remained in stable condition during the entire forty-five-minute operation. The surgeon explained when the drill penetrated the brain cavity, spinal fluid shot nearly three feet into the air. Relieved and feeling as if I had survived death myself, I asked when we could see him.

As with any operation, Isaac was heavily sedated and in recovery. The surgeon expected within a few hours he would be stabilized and moved back to a hospital room. Although the danger of losing Isaac had temporarily passed, the surgeon cautioned more surgery would be required to remove the tumor. In addition, an aggressive schedule of cancer treatments would follow.

Isaac came back to the room heavily sedated with a tube draining fluid off his brain. It would be the next day before he was fully conscious and awake. Collapsing from exhaustion, I fell asleep wondering what tomorrow would bring.

A Cell Phone Ringing

R arely in Oklahoma is there snow on the ground on Christmas day. This year would be no exception as the landscape outside was a golden amber brown. The bite of a cold north wind made sitting near the wood stove a pleasant reminder it was still the holidays. As a small child, Christmas was my favorite holiday and time of the year. I loved the candy and the toys. As I grew older, I found myself most happy to be around family and friends on this special day. Unlike a child, I also enjoyed sleeping in a little late on Christmas day.

Isaac and Caleb had gone to bed way past their normal bedtimes. Both were entering the teenage years and the chance to stay up late during Christmas break was a present in itself. Recently gone with the ages of our kids were the childhood traditions of Christmas. Cookies on the fireplace mantel and milk left out for Santa Claus were replaced with a new custom - a scavenger hunt.

Both boys awoke to an envelope taped to their nightstands with their first hint. Racing to get dressed they set out to find the gift left for them by "Santa," which in all fairness was left by Dacia. A series of clues would lead Caleb to the dryer where his PlayStation 2 was found. Running into the family room, I remember him yelling - "I got a PS2." Isaac seemed a little upset as his clues led him to the Christmas tree. Feeling as if he had been cheated by his brother's gift, he was baffled when he heard a cell phone ringing. He noticed it was coming from somewhere behind the tree. Picking up the phone and holding it to his ear, he heard us say from the other room, "Merry Christmas Isaac." In Isaac's mind he had arrived at adulthood. He now had his own personal cell phone - an LG slider!

It would be only a few months later this very cell phone would remind me of how precious life is.

A Day the World Returned to Normal

I saac slept well thanks to the narcotic pain medications administered throughout the night. Dacia had gone home to gather a few belongings in preparation for a long hospital stay. I found myself staring at all the medical equipment, anxious about what would happen when Isaac awakened. Sitting there, watching him asleep, I found myself hungry for the first time in two days. Before leaving for the cafeteria I spoke with the nurse about calling me should the surgeon come by the room. I expected it would be quiet as the anesthesia drugs from surgery had been slow to wear off.

I arrived back on the floor in time to be greeted by our neurosurgeon. He stopped me to discuss the upcoming tumor resection surgery. He told me Isaac would undergo a brain MRI early in the morning which would determine the exact size and location of the tumor. Surgery was planned for the next day at 6:00 AM.

Despite the first successful operation, he cautioned this second surgery would determine the extent of any brain damage and the type of cancer to be treated. I wondered how much Isaac remembered prior to surgery? Did he know why he was here? Did he grasp the gravity of the situation before him? Quickly something caught the corner of my eye as my conversation with the surgeon came to an end. The TV was on in the room, and waiting for me on the other side of the door was a wide-awake child who called me by name when he saw me in the hall.

I was pleasantly surprised when I stepped into the room. Isaac was awake and appeared happy. He looked up and said, "Hi dad, can I have bacon and eggs for breakfast? Can Caleb come up and play his PS2 with me? Also, can you tell mom to bring my cell phone from home?" My thoughts drifted back to a few months ago on Christmas Day when he received the phone. In a surreal moment it was as if the world had returned to normal, if not for just one day.

Learning to Eat Again

T he operation began promptly at 6:00 AM just as the surgeon said. Unlike the previous surgery two days prior, a large gathering of extended family and friends filled the waiting room. A nurse diligently called the landline phone at the top of every hour. She gave very few details, but her reassuring words lifted my spirits during the difficult five-hour operation.

Usually our family gatherings were loud and filled with laughter. Today, among those who had assembled the mood was restrained and serious. I did not know it at the time, but my brothers had brought dress suits with them on their trip to Tulsa in the event Isaac's surgery ended in a funeral. Feeling helpless and powerless to control the outcome before me, I closed my eyes and listened for the phone to ring. Somewhat stunned, my younger brother Matt nudged me and said something which brought a tear to my eye. He had just got off the phone with a Captain at the Greeley *(Colorado)* Police Department. Matt was a detective and was keeping his boss informed of our situation. He said, "My Captain is going to send Isaac a gold medal service coin. It's reserved for officers who show heroic acts of bravery and courage. He felt Isaac had earned his rank among Greeley's finest." Immediately, I was taken back in time to the day we met with a fertility specialist. Isaac's coming into this world was compared to the swipe of a gold coin. For a short time, thinking about this gold coin gave me an inner peace and a sense of courage.

It was going on noon and the phone had not rang. A nurse came to the lobby and asked us to follow her to a consult room to meet the surgeon. Although the danger of losing Isaac in surgery was not a concern, the mood was serious and grim. The surgeon told us the malignant softball size tumor he removed was situated near the brain stem. The tumor had literally attached itself to the spinal cord and about a sugar cube size amount remained. The massive tumor had caused damage to the cerebellum lobe of the brain which controls balance and fine motor skills. Notwithstanding, the area of the spinal cord where the tumor was found controlled eyesight and facial movements. It would not be until the next day when Isaac was awake could the damage be fully assessed.

Isaac was moved to a pediatric ICU room and listed in critical condition. Although the risk of infection was low; blood pressure, fever and heart rate were of grave concern throughout the night. The next morning the surgeon arrived before dawn. He ordered the nurses to place blankets over the windows to darken the room. He told us Isaac would have severe sensitivity to light and to expect significant impairment in his fine motor skills. He compared his recovery to an older adult recovering from a stroke. However, Isaac's brain was young and still growing. Different lobes of his teenage brain could restore some of the fine motor skills the tumor had taken away. This became firmly evident when he attempted to walk as his ghastly gait reminded me of a two-year old trying to stand for the first time. Further, Isaac began to cry when he attempted to unwrap a popsicle. Giving assistance, I placed it in his hand *(he gripped it like a stick)* only to notice he lifted it towards his ear. Realizing a brazen new reality, I surmised Isaac would need lessons on learning to eat again.

Looming on the horizon was a more pressing concern - cancer. This disease would bring our family to its knees and leave Isaac clinging to the hope of a normal life beyond a wounded warrior. Life as we knew it would never be the same.

"I Would Go to St. Jude"

The oncology team at the hospital scheduled a meeting with us to discuss cancer treatments at 4:00 PM. We decided it would be best to meet in a private consultation area and not directly involve Isaac in the conversation. The oncologist's treatment plan brought more heartache and pain. Isaac would require six months of outpatient radiation directed to the center of his brain. The high grade of radiation would leave him with significant cognitive impairments. The doctor compared his intellectual level of functioning after treatment to a retarded child. Further, three chemotherapy drugs administered over eight cycles roughly one month apart would require isolation and hospitalization. The powerful cancer fighting drugs would cause complete hearing loss and nerve damage in his legs. If Isaac were to survive, he would be rendered to a wheelchair, deaf, and left with severe brain damage. The oncologist told us the survival rate for his type of cancer was only thirty-nine percent. In utter disbelief I painfully asked, "You mean after fourteen months of treatment, the best you can do is give me back my child with no quality of life and very little chance of survival?" Her compassionate response was pointed and direct, "Mr. Walsh, I have been an oncologist at this hospital for twenty-five years, this is the third worst case of cancer we have ever seen."

The doctor continued by saying there was another option to consider. A research scientist from St. Jude Children's Research Hospital had called after reviewing Isaac's diagnosis posted to the cancer registry database at the Centers for Disease Control *(CDC)*. Isaac met the criteria for a pediatric clinical trial being done in Memphis, Tennessee. The treatment plan would involve six weeks of experimental radiation to the brain and spine. In addition, the second phase of the trial would involve taking the same three chemotherapy drugs used in standard treatment but given at a much higher dose. The high levels of toxicity would bring him to the verge of death and risk major organ failure. In order to survive, Isaac would be infused with stem cells harvested from his own bone marrow. In all, he would undergo four rounds of chemotherapy roughly one month apart. She said there was significant risk of complications including death due to the experimental nature of the aggressive treatment. However, it came with an eighty-five percent survival rate for those who made it to the end.

Contemplating the two options before us, the doctor began to break down when I asked, "What would you do if it were your child?" Unable to contain her reserved emotions, tears began to fill her eyes as I heard her say, "Isaac is young and does not have any underlying health problems, he has a better chance than most of making it to the end. If it were my child, I would go to St. Jude."

On the morning of March 11, 2011 we signed the consent forms for Isaac to become a St. Jude patient. We also gave our permission for the cancerous tumor to be shipped Priority Alert FedEx to the neuro-oncology research team at St. Jude in Memphis, Tennessee.

Team Isaac

B asketball practice had ended early and the damp cold of winter made the thought of eating out appealing. Like most young kids going to McDonalds was the highlight of their day but much to the chagrin of mine. As Isaac and Caleb scurried off to the play area, I noticed a decorated jar collecting coins for the Ronald McDonald Foundation next to the cash register. Pictured on the side of the jar was a cancer-stricken child with no hair. I deposited coins into the vase naively thinking nothing like this could ever happen to my child. However, it would be only a few months later when Isaac's picture would be placed around our town. A "TEAM," had been formed by our friends in the community to show their support for a young life in crisis.

My wife and I were educators in a small bedroom community in the Tulsa *(Oklahoma)* metropolitan area back in 2011. Teachers working in small communities often become well known due to their work with children. My work as a principal had afforded me the opportunity to become acquainted with several of our local business leaders and school board members. Dacia taught elementary school and through the years watched many of her students grow up to become government officials, working professionals and parents themselves. Our family resembled the traditional middle-class American household with two working professional parents and a pair of young children who were active in sports.

Isaac's cancer diagnosis caught our close-knit community off guard. Many in our inner circle of friends expressed deep sorrow and were stunned at the news one of the Walsh boys had brain cancer. Family members were overwhelmed with

21

grief upon hearing of our calamity. Our church shared in our pain and wanted to show their support for our family. Many began wearing a "TEAM Isaac," blue bracelet to show their solidarity with our desire to see Isaac get well. Another group printed t-shirts in an effort to raise both an awareness of Isaac's illness and fundraise to support our stay in Memphis. Countless other events were done to support our family during this perilous time. Each time, Dacia and I were at a loss for words to express our heartfelt thanks and appreciation for the tremendous show of support bestowed upon our family.

There were some who gave more than just money. Some invested their time to support our long stay in Memphis. My next-door neighbor Erik Noleen organized an effort to keep our 1.5-acre lawn mowed throughout the summer, and leaves picked up in the fall. Erik and his wife Linda bought Isaac an iPad which was easier for him to use than a cell phone due to a loss of fine motor control in his hands immediately following his surgery. My dad diligently watered our shrubbery during the Oklahoma drought of 2011, and kept our house in good working order. Notwithstanding, neighbors George and Sandy Pinkstaff stopped by daily to pick up and sort our mail. Due to making monthly trips back to Tulsa, we never had our mail forwarded to Memphis. In all, we never had to worry about taking care of our home during the entire time we were away.

Looking back our family and friends gave us the financial and logistical support needed to take care of Isaac four hundred miles from home. We never had to bear the burden of hiring people to care for our lawn, check on our house, or care for family pets. As I reflect back to this time, I'm reminded of the goodness of mankind in tumultuous times. I believe within all of us there is a desire to make the world a better place - for the downtrodden and those who feel defeated by the undeserved tragedies of life.

Every family facing a critical health crisis is met with the anxiety of how this stressful event will impact members of the immediate family. Our eleven-year-old son Caleb was thriving in fifth grade, or so we thought. His teacher told us Caleb became very quiet in class and at times did not complete his homework which was rare for him. In his own way, Caleb began to process the thought of losing his brother at a very young age. He would be left heartbroken seeing the taillights of our car pull out of the driveway on our way to the airport, not knowing if he would ever see his older brother again.

We struggled with leaving him behind. He was only eleven years old and did not understand the gravity of the situation before us. Caleb would repeatedly beg us to bring him to Memphis. In anguish, Dacia would wrestle with the cost of separating him from us during this critical time in our lives. Her concerns centered around the long-term effect of separating him from his family when he needed them the most. However, the risks posed by bringing him to a place where Isaac would require strict isolation and spend weeks at a time in a hospital would prove futile. The best we could do would be to make frequent trips to Oklahoma. Then when appropriate bring him to Memphis for a visit.

Soon we would pack up our TEAM Isaac t-shirts and wear our colorful blue bracelets as we headed east. It would be a lonely journey as we didn't know anyone in the large metropolitan area of Memphis, Tennessee. However, it would change once we walked through the gates of St. Jude Children's Research Hospital.

Part II

A New Beginning
St. Jude Children's Research Hospital

Finding Cures. Saving Children.

S ituated in Memphis, Tennessee a few blocks from the mighty Mississippi River is the large sprawling campus of St. Jude Children's Research Hospital. Founded by legendary entertainer Danny Thomas, the hospital garners its name from St. Jude Thaddeus also known as the patron saint of hopeless causes. Much like those who walked through its doors, Danny Thomas struggled early in life.

As an expectant struggling father trying to gain a foothold in the entertainment industry in the early 1950's, in a Detroit church a despondent Thomas made a vow to the Patron Saint by praying, "Show me my way in life and I will build you a shrine." Soon thereafter, Danny Thomas became a household name on radio, in film and on television, He kept his solemn promise when St. Jude opened its doors to cancer-stricken children on February 4, 1962. Believing no child should die in the dawn of life, Danny Thomas embarked on a journey that would bring thousands of doctors, nurses and scientists from all over the world together, with the sole mission of finding cures and saving children.

Unlike most hospitals, St. Jude treats only pediatric cancer and other life-threatening diseases. Children are admitted when they meet the protocols of a research study being done on their type of cancer and/or disease. The hospital itself has only seventy-eight beds but accommodates roughly eight thousand patients annually with most treated on an outpatient basis. There are some children whose treatment protocols require a long-term stay in Memphis. For them, housing is provided in an apartment style living arrangement at the Ronald McDonald House or the St. Jude Target House. Lastly, St. Jude has been recognized by US World and News Report as the nation's top hospital for treating pediatric cancer.

As for me, I came with my family to St. Jude on March 30, 2011 in hopes of becoming a part of the miracles made possible by one man's vision, to save the lives of children. The time had come for Isaac's cancer treatments to begin.

A Place of Hope and Healing

My first glimpse of St. Jude would later mirror my impression of its employees, I was awestruck by the beautiful flowers and immaculate grounds. Embolden on the side of the building was the image of a praying child which I came to realize was the trademark image of St. Jude. As our driver Charles brought us to the main hospital lobby, I noticed a large gold dome which prominently staked out the memorial grounds of the hospital's founder Danny Thomas. Three times during Isaac's course of treatment in Memphis, I would reverently sit in this beautiful garden contemplating life without him as he nearly succumbed to cancer.

Dacia recalled her first memory of St. Jude, etched in her mind were parents pulling children in wagons, older kids in wheelchairs, and some children walking with the aid of prosthetic limbs. Dacia also remembered Isaac's first words when walking through the large turnstile doors. She heard him say, "It's not fair these kids are so sick." Dacia felt a sense of sadness as it appeared the worst cases of cancer from around the world came to St. Jude. However, this would change soon after meeting the oncology team who would be in charge of Isaac's treatment plan.

Thousands of children diagnosed with cancer had come before us. In our clinical trial which started in 2003, Isaac would be among the first five-hundred children treated. Waiting in an exam room, we were greeted by the neuro-oncology team which would later become like family. I immediately became impressed when I met the St. Jude Chair of Pediatric Neuro-Oncology, Dr. Amar Gajjar. An immigrant doctor from India, Dr. Gajjar served as the chief investigator for the clinical trial. Further, Dr. Gajjar had published research on this type of cancer and was considered the world's foremost expert on treating this type of childhood brain tumor. His assistant and serving as our primary neuro-oncologist was Dr. Giles Robinson who hailed from upstate New York and was a Boston College graduate. Dr. Robinson was currently conducting a molecular study on Isaac's type of cancer. He was already in possession of Isaac's tumor tissue as it had been shipped overnight via FedEx from Tulsa when we signed to become a St Jude patient.

Dr. Robinson asked for signed consent as he wanted to complete a DNA study of Isaac's blood to better determine what drugs would be used during treatment. In all, we gave permission for St. Jude to conduct fourteen research studies on Isaac. The studies would include psychology, nutrition, sleep disorders, genome project mapping, life skills, brain functioning MRI experimental study and school adaptation to name just a few.

After a long day of travel and medical appointments I was exhausted. I did not need any urging about going to bed. As I closed my eyes, I felt a sense of release. My thoughts were no longer tethered to a rope leading to a cistern of death and despair. Rather, I had become a member of the St. Jude family. It was an invitation no parent ever wanted. However, it was the first time since our cancer journey began in which I realized we had arrived at a place of hope and healing.

"All a Family Should Worry About is Helping Their Child Live"

D anny Thomas realized in the early 1950's he would need the help of the business community to fulfill his vision of opening a hospital. Racing across the nation with his wife Rose Marie to solicit donations and enlisting the help of local Memphis business leaders, Mr. Thomas was able to raise enough funding to secure the building of the hospital. Notwithstanding, Danny Thomas knew additional money would be needed to fund the annual operation of the clinic. Calling upon an immigrant group of like-minded Arab American business leaders, Danny Thomas convened a conference in Chicago in 1957. Emerging from their discussion was a commitment to honor their forefathers by creating a charitable organization to raise funds for the hospital's yearly budget and to ensure no family would ever receive a bill for treatment received at St. Jude. Tracing its beginnings to this conference, The American Lebanese Syrian Associated Charities (ALSAC) was formed. Today, ALSAC is the second largest medical charitable organization in the world. The charity raises over $1 billion dollars annually to support cancer research and pay not only the medical bills for all St. Jude patients but their living expenses as well. However, when I first arrived at St. Jude, I did not realize all medical expenses would be covered, due to a commitment Danny Thomas made almost fifty years ago.

It was four days after we had arrived at the hospital when I finally found time to open a large stack of mail I had brought from home. I was dismayed when I read a letter from our medical insurance company. The correspondence stated due to joining a pediatric clinical trial at an out of network hospital, all treatment performed at St. Jude would not be covered by our insurance plan. In disbelief and bewilderment, I asked the next day during registration to speak with our patient care representative. We had met Joyce on our first day during our hospital tour, and her wonderful advice would be something I would rely on for years to come. I told her our insurance company would not cover Isaac's cancer treatment at St. Jude and I needed to speak with someone about making payment arrangements. Her polite reply came with a beaming smile, "Mr. Walsh, you will never receive a bill from St. Jude. All a family should worry about is helping their child live."

Two Steps Back

I remember staring at the lovely flowers and hearing the sounds of birds chirping in the garden marking the burial site of Danny Thomas. The gold dome and graveside memorial of the hospital's founder came to represent a place of solitude and solace for me. I had come to the St. Jude Pavilion to reflect on the sobering news we had just received from our radiation oncologist. Dr. Larry Kun spearheaded one of the most successful pediatric brain tumor radiation treatment programs in the country. His counsel was direct and compassionate, but it also brought back memories of what we had heard in Tulsa. Isaac's tumor had started growing again. Due to having a residual amount of cancerous tissue, the experimental radiation would be delivered to his entire spine and a boost of high-grade radiation would go to the center of his brain. The side effects were even more concerning: significant cognitive impairments marked by an IQ deficit of at least twenty points, and damage to the endocrine system. Isaac would require a multiple disabilities class should he return to school and would need assistance for daily living throughout adulthood. The aftereffects of radiation would not be seen for months after treatment and would come with lifelong disabilities.

Listening to the wind rustling the leaves in the garden during the late afternoon brought back tearful memories. Reflecting on Isaac's life as a young adolescent child who just now was beginning to understand the world around him brought even more pain. Allowing him to undergo this radiation treatment would change his life forever. In some respects, I felt as if we were leading him into a tunnel opening to a new standard of affliction and impediments I would not even want for myself. In essence, I felt as if we had taken two giant steps back. However, the next morning we were introduced to a St Jude neurosurgeon who would not only save Isaac's life three times during our ten-month stay in Memphis but transform the entire trajectory of cancer treatment at St. Jude.

St. Jude Neurosurgeon Dr. Paul Klimo

D r. Paul Klimo is a St. Jude surgeon who had been tested by the battle lines of war. Entering the United States Air Force after completing a long history of medical training is not the path every surgeon takes to begin their career. However, five years after American Forces invaded Afghanistan in 2006, Dr. Klimo entered active military service and was stationed at Wright-Patterson Air Force Base near Dayton, Ohio.

Dr. Klimo answered the most heroic call of all when his unit known as the 88th Medical Wing was deployed to Bagram Airfield in Afghanistan during Operation Enduring Freedom. Utilizing his talents with only basic medical equipment on the battlefield, Dr. Klimo and his team completed over three-hundred surgeries on both wounded American troops and Afghan civilians who were caught in the crossfire of war. His surgeries would include fifty-seven Afghani children who were brought to American bases by their parents in search of a miracle to save their young lives. Lastly, Dr. Klimo served four years with the United States Air Force and received an honorable discharge in 2010 as a Lt. Colonel-Select. As for me, I met Dr. Klimo in hopes of removing all the cancer from Isaac's brain which would allow for a lower grade of radiation and thus possibly spare him from severe cognitive impairments.

Initially, our first three weeks at St. Jude were filled with medical tests, research study consent appointments and visits with our primary oncologists who would coordinate Isaac's care. One day in early April, Dr. Robinson told us Isaac's case was being referred to neurosurgery. Despite already having had two surgeries in an attempt to remove the tumor, he wanted us to visit with a St. Jude neurosurgeon named Dr. Paul Klimo. I will never forget the day I had the pleasure to meet this heroic veteran and the man who would six months later save Isaac's life. Dr. Paul Klimo was a young and slender man who showed tremendous compassion for our family. He spoke in clear layman's terms about how he felt a third surgery might help Isaac. Dr. Klimo explained the operating room at St. Jude was one of only a dozen hospitals in the United States that possessed the next generation MRI imaging equipment which made the risk of performing a third surgery on Isaac a proposal to seriously consider. He compared the high definition MRI scans at St. Jude to those of an antiquated bubble TV image found at our hospital back in Tulsa. Further, Dr. Klimo believed more of the tumor could be removed using a high-tech device known as an "Intraoperative MRI." This apparatus would allow him to cut tumor tissue off the spinal cord and see in real time if all the cancerous tissue had been removed. If successful, this surgery could change the total trajectory of treatment at St. Jude.

Shortly after our visit, we signed the surgery consent papers for the operation. Due to time being of the essence, the surgeon scheduled the procedure two days after our initial meeting.

A Ten-Hour Surgery
Which Changed Our World

L e Bonheur Children's Hospital is a sister facility of St. Jude. Isaac's surgery would be at this nearby trauma center with Dr. Klimo performing the operation. The surgery preop area resembled something I would picture at a children's play museum. Toys, beautiful murals and cartoon characters were in abundance, however, the bite of the cold air-conditioned room reminded me of what we had come for – surgery.

The surgery carried considerable risk due the cancer's location on the brain stem. Infection and failure of a nonprogrammable shunt draining fluid off the brain were a concern due to the nature of removing a cancerous mass from an area of hemorrhaging tissue. In addition, the location in which the surgeon would be operating was the site where the optic nerves connected to the spinal cord – blindness was a pressing worry. Dr. Klimo had a calmness and presence which settled my apprehension and uneasiness. Unlike the previous surgery in Tulsa only three weeks prior, today's surgery was being performed by a battle tested warrior and one of the world's foremost experts on this type of tumor removal.

We had barely settled into the family waiting area when a young nurse came to move us to a neuro intensive care unit recovery room. Dr. Klimo expected the surgery to last the better part of the day and thought a hospital room would prove more comfortable. Much can be written of what a person thinks about when their child is undergoing major brain surgery. As for me, I struggled to focus on reading a book and watching TV. My thoughts were erratic and speckled with tinges of worry as I contemplated the ongoing operation. It was as if the earth stood still while Isaac lay in a nearby operating room for ten hours, with a surgeon delicately cutting cancerous tissue off his brain stem and spinal cord. Predictably fighting off the urge to fall asleep, I immediately sat up when Dr. Klimo appeared in the hallway outside our room. The surgeon's words brought sighs of relief when he told us all the cancer had been removed.

Throughout the surgery the intraoperative MRI machine was used to run three scans - each time allowing the surgeon to cut deeper into the spinal cord to remove the malignant tissue. Isaac's optic nerve on the left side was severely swollen, however a full recovery was expected as the nerve remained intact and was not permanently damaged. The successful operation came at a price however, the seventh nerve which controls facial movements on the left side of the face had been severed. Isaac's appearance on his left cheek was marked by a significant "droop," much like that of an elderly stroke victim. Like any typical teenager, it was difficult for Isaac to comprehend the tradeoff of a maligned appearance vs. a cancer free scan.

I realized this ten-hour surgery would change our world for years to come. Radiation could be altered to a lower grade and would no longer cause significant brain damage. Isaac would now have a fighting chance to reclaim a small part of the life he once knew.

A Long Road to Recovery

A few days later we met with Dr. Robinson who gave us the official good news, the radiation grade could be decreased to a lower level. The neuro-oncology team all agreed Isaac could be placed into a lower risk group in the clinical trial; the expected cognitive impairments could for the most part be avoided. I was naïve thinking Isaac would be relieved to hear this seemingly good news. He was dejected and would often cry when looking at himself in a mirror. Cancer carries life and death consequences but for Isaac, a deformed face was worse than the distant thought of having brain damage later in life. At the time, even I struggled with trying to make him understand how critical it was for the radiation grade to be lowered to a "safer," level.

Isaac would refuse to talk about his feelings. I was worried he might become angry and bitter towards us because of his contorted face. We accepted counseling from the psychology department, as this was a part of the comprehensive approach to cancer management at St. Jude.

Another pressing concern was our youngest son Caleb. He too was struggling with the thought of losing his older brother. Caleb became increasingly concerned he might also have brain cancer. He would often complain of headaches at school and wanted to come and stay with us in Memphis. The logistics of removing him from school and taking care of him under very difficult circumstances in a hospital setting nearly four hundred miles from our home, rendered this scenario impossible. We considered asking for a CT scan of his brain to ease his concerns but decided against it due to exposing him to needless radiation. Selfishly, I did not want to give credibility to his worst fears. However, Dacia and I decided early on we would make trips back to Sapulpa to be with Caleb when Isaac was no longer hospitalized. Reminding Caleb of our love for him during this difficult time was just as important as providing Isaac with the parental support he would need to survive.

As for me, I found an inner peace by starting a social media Caring Bridge site to update family and friends. Whenever Isaac was hospitalized I would update the site twice daily. The daily condolences, comforting words and tributes of our extended family and friends afforded me hope and strength. The daily routine of tests and appointments was about to soon change – the time to begin the first phase of the clinical trial was now upon us.

Part III
SJMB03 St. Jude Pediatric Cancer Clinical Trial

Experimental Radiation

D r. Larry Kun would serve as chief radiation oncologist for the first part of the clinical trial. He oversaw one of the largest pediatric radiation oncology programs in the country and was considered an expert in this type of treatment. We found him to be very friendly and welcoming from the first day we met him. Dr. Kun told us about his own children which included their favorite places to eat in Memphis. He suggested we try Huey's Hamburgers, which quickly became one of our most cherished places to eat while in Memphis - for years to come. Dr. Kun's unique ability to interact with patients and his expertise in the medical field led to a series of promotions where he became the hospital's Clinical Director and later Executive Vice-President. St. Jude suffered an enormous loss when Dr. Larry Kun succumbed to cancer on May 27, 2018. He will be remembered by many for his kindness and medical expertise. As for me, I will always reverently think of him as the one who guided us during our first phase of treatment.

The radiation was considered experimental in nature because the laser beam went to all areas of the body where spinal fluid was found. Although Isaac had no tumors in the spinal cord, the entire spine and brain would receive radiation to prevent a breakaway cancerous cell from later becoming active. In all, Isaac received thirty-one treatments of radiation. Due to the location of the cancerous tissue on the brain stem, a boost of radiation was sent to this area to prevent any future growth of cancerous tissue at the site of the tumor.

Isaac was considered old enough to lay still for roughly twenty minutes during the radiation therapy. However, younger children had to be put under anesthesia each morning prior to the start of the treatment. Thus, almost all of Isaac's treatments were in the afternoon which allowed the "fasting," younger kids to go first. Prior to starting the radiation therapy, a team of St. Jude professionals created a mold of Isaac's face while lying face down. The goalie hockey type mask would serve as a brace to secure his head in a permanent position, to deliver pinpoint radiation to the site of the tumor. Doctors tattooed some small dark brown lines on his neck and back which would serve as guideposts to line up the radiation beams each time a treatment was given. Initially, the side effects associated with radiation were just fatigue and tiredness. However, about one week into treatment everything began to change.

"Why Are All Cancer Kids Bald?"

T he sound of someone moving about in the bathroom caught my attention. Normally, Isaac slept in late as he was never known to be a morning person. However, this morning was different. When I entered the bathroom, Isaac was clearly upset as I could see tears streaming down his cheeks. His question forced upon me a deep sense of sadness as there was nothing I could do to spare him of what was about to happen. I could see the suffering in his eyes when he asked, "Dad, why are all cancer kids bald?" I noticed in the shower clumps of hair lay littered across the base of the tub. As expected, the radiation had caused the hair follicles to die and thus large chunks of hair began falling out after one week of treatment. Isaac would cling to a patchwork of hair for only one day, for by evening the slightest touch of the hand upended the hair strands like petting a shedding dog.

At the time I wore my hair very short, and while at St. Jude I used a pair of barber shears to keep it trimmed. One of my saddest days was having to take the hair clippers and cut Isaac's hair thus leaving him bald. I remember telling him, "Isaac, it's not just cancer kids who are bald. There is the dad of a cancer child who is bald too!" Shortly thereafter, I took a razor and shaved my head in a show of allegiance to my son, in saying we would get through this together. It's a pledge I keep to this day.

Isaac would struggle with a loss of hair for the entire ten months we were at St. Jude. He wore a hat to cover the large surgery scars and hide the shiny white scalp the radiation left behind. On one hand, I did notice a growing acceptance on his part while in the confines of St. Jude, as most of the kids at the hospital had lost their hair. Boys and girls alike shared a common bond as nobody seemed to notice their distorted appearance. However, returning to a normal world became difficult as Isaac would try to shut out a cruel society, which stared at his scars and looked twice when he took off his hat.

Not all strangers viewed life through a gawking set of discriminatory glasses. One day in early May, Isaac and I went to a Triple-A Memphis Redbirds baseball game. Before the game started Isaac had gone to the bathroom and lost his hat. Returning to his seat, he became anxious and upset as his appearance was now out in the open for all to see. I did my best to calm him down and told him we would go get another. A stranger behind me motioned for me to stay with Isaac at our seat. A few minutes later a man and his wife came back with an expensive fitted Memphis Redbirds ball cap and a pair of sunglasses. I will never forget the smile on Isaac's face when he put on the hat and sunglasses, once again he was a normal child in a judgmental world. This simple random act of kindness by a discerning man and his wife, reminded me the goodness of mankind transcends a society unaware their stares bring pain to those whose lives are marred by the side effects of cancer.

Reality Begins

At the onset of radiation, we noticed extreme fatigue as Isaac would sleep most of the afternoon and take long naps on the weekends. This was to be expected according to Dr. Kun. Outdistancing the exhaustion was Isaac's recovery from four major brain surgeries over the course of just thirty days. Due to poor balance, reduced fine motor skills, and weakened muscles in his extremities – Isaac had a daily regime of physical and occupational therapy sessions. These sessions were difficult for him. Prior to his cancer diagnosis, he was a little league all-star athlete. I vividly remember a day when Isaac was attempting to shoot a basketball during a physical therapy session with his therapist Terry. It was humbling and difficult to watch as just three months prior Isaac was sinking three-point shots in his seventh-grade basketball games. A few months later at St. Jude he was ghostly white and bald. His movements were uncoordinated and erratic. Unable to tightly grip the ball due to poor coordination, Isaac began to cry as the basketball would slip from his shaking hands. Gently placing the basketball in his fingers and demonstrating how to properly shoot the ball only brought about more tears. In some respects, there was a part of me which changed too. Never again would I attempt to show him the athletic life he left behind. Rather, my focus would be on restoring his ability to face each new day with a determined attitude void of failure and ridicule. The life he once knew as an athlete had gone by the wayside. More so, my societal view as a father playing catch with his son in the backyard was now in my distant past. A new reality set in as cancer had changed both our lives forever.

Aside from the recovery from surgery was the issue of Isaac's drooping face. The sagging facial muscles created problems with speech and swallowing. Isaac had been assigned a speech pathologist who would seek to circumvent the regular patterns of chewing food and allow him to compensate for the loss of movements in his left cheek. St. Jude speech pathologist Angela Eftink had a pleasant demeanor about her which quickly won Isaac over. She was genuine and possessed personality traits like those of the best teachers I had met throughout my tenure as a principal in a public school. Not realizing it at the time, I later learned Mrs. Eftink worked part-time in a nearby elementary school as a speech pathologist.

Isaac's speech therapy sessions would challenge us. In the beginning of our time at St. Jude, Isaac would cling to our presence during appointments. His behavior was reminiscent of when he was four years old after being left with a babysitter. On his first day of speech therapy with Angela something was different. Isaac asked if he could go to speech class with Angela alone. I did not want to let him, yet reserved of emotion, I watched as a large wooden door with a small window closed behind him. Isaac disappeared into a long hallway in which every door looked the same. Forty-five minutes later he returned with Angela to the lobby. His smile resembled a bent kinked line as only one side of his face would move. He had begun to gain the confidence needed to endure his greatest battle - to eliminate cancer from his young body. The next phase of the clinical trial would be marked by several encounters with death, and the greatest sickness ever clinically imposed by mankind.

Preparation for Chemotherapy

I often tell people Isaac's radiation therapy brought me to my knees. In truth, the experimental chemotherapy thrust me face first to the ground drowning in my tears, as I contemplated life without my first-born son. In this experimental part of the trial, Isaac would be administered three chemotherapy drugs *(Vincristine, cisplatin and cyclophosphamide)* via an IV drip at double their standard dose. Due to the high levels of toxicity, major organ failure and death were a serious concern. For him to survive, he would be infused with his own stem cells. In preparation for this phase of the trial to begin, several new medical procedures had to take place.

First, Isaac had to undergo minor surgery to have a double Hickman line *(similar to a chemo port)* placed in his chest. It would be through this device Isaac would receive liquid nutrition which would be prepared in a pharmacy according to his blood test results. The Total Parental Nutrition (TPN) would be administered throughout the day and replaced by IV fluids overnight. Dacia and I would undertake lessons on disinfecting the lines and hooking up the various bags of fluids. Further, we took turns sleeping in his room as he needed assistance to go to the bathroom at night. Due to the careful analysis of his blood labs, Isaac never lost a pound during the six-month chemotherapy protocol, despite eating less than one child's dinner portion of food the entire time.

Secondly, stem cell therapy was considered experimental by our medical insurance company but lifesaving cutting-edge research by St. Jude. Isaac's cancer was found in his spinal fluid and thus the bone marrow stem cells found in the blood stream were not contaminated by the cancer cells. In order to harvest the cells, Isaac received injections in an area under both arms for fourteen days to stimulate the growth of the stem cells in his bloodstream. On day fifteen, Isaac underwent surgery to place a large dialysis type line into an artery in his leg which would allow his blood to be filtered through a machine. In all, the filtering process took forty-eight hours. Having collected billions of stem cells, St. Jude would freeze and place them in a secure area to have on hand for the chemo cycles in the months to come.

Lastly, the radiation caused concern over Isaac's MRI brain scans. An edema *(sack of fluid)* had formed at the site of the tumor. Numerous tests had to be done to determine if the swelling would cause neurological problems once the onset of chemotherapy started. In the end, the team of neurosurgeons believed the swelling was a result of the residual scar tissue, thus the final part of the trial could commence.

"I'm at Chesapeake Arena"

The experimental nature of the trial would involve four chemo cycles. On the first day of the trial, three chemotherapy drugs were administered via an IV drip. Due to Isaac's immune system bottoming out at zero, stem cells were given on day seven to prevent his major organs from failing and thus allowing him the ability to survive. If all went well, his immune system blood markers would recover to a healthy level by day fourteen and another round could proceed approximately two weeks later. Surprisingly, the first course of treatment was much like the onset of radiation – fatigue, tiredness, lack of appetite and pain. Looming on the horizon only sixteen days later was another chemo round.

At the time, we felt comfortable with Dacia going back to Sapulpa to visit Caleb. At a very young age, Caleb excelled at every sport he tried. His ability to run had caught the eye of the high school cross country coaches. Soon thereafter, Caleb began competing in cross country meets on the weekends with the Sapulpa team in the elementary age group. His prowess and talents had won him a collection of medals and trophies. More so, his athletic ability gave him an outlet to deal with the pain of his family leaving him behind.

Isaac and I settled into our apartment at the St. Jude Target House in Memphis after being discharged from the hospital. Around midnight I could hear Isaac coughing and gagging. I quickly noticed he was vomiting all over the bed. Isaac was listless and confused, I had seen Dr. Giles administer his neurological exams long enough to know something was seriously wrong. Finding a wheelchair in the hallway, I gently rolled Isaac to the car where I lifted him into the front seat. Thirty minutes later Isaac was admitted to St. Jude where a CT scan revealed his brain was swollen twice its normal size. The next morning Isaac was transported by an ambulance to Le Bonheur Children's Hospital which is where many St. Jude neuro surgeries are performed.

By the time Dacia arrived, after a long six-hour drive from Oklahoma, Isaac was awaiting surgery in a preop room. He was unconscious and his vital signs suddenly began dropping. His heart rate and blood pressure were dangerously low as his swollen brain started to shut his body down. Fear set in as I watched Isaac's lifeless body transition to the stillness and eerie peace marked only by the onset of death. I could hear a team of doctors coming down the hall. Swiftly, a young female surgeon placed a long needle into the reservoir hole which had been drilled into his skull while in Tulsa. Drawing two vials of spinal fluid off his brain, Isaac's fingers slowly began to show movement, and his eyes gently started to open. In a hurried effort to determine if he had suffered any brain damage, I asked Isaac if he knew what happened and where he was. His response brought a puzzled and quizzical look from the surgeon but a smile from me when he said, "I'm at Chesapeake Arena." The doctor appeared dumbfounded and more than likely had never heard anything like this before. For me however, it was pure Isaac as I told the doctor, "It's the home arena of the NBA Oklahoma City Thunder – I'll take it. He's back!"

My joyous moment was soon tampered by a new reality when the surgeon explained the spinal fluid pulled off the brain marked approximately two hours before death would make an attempt to take Isaac again. Surgery would start in less than one hour.

Death Came Calling at 3:00 AM

D r. Klimo was paged to perform the fifth brain surgery on Isaac which by my count had occurred in less than two months. The CT scans were inconclusive as to the reason for the swelling of Isaac's brain. The goal of the procedure was to install a drain line in the reservoir opening to utilize the pull of gravity, and thus reduce the enlargement of the brain. It was a rather quick operation which lasted only forty-five minutes. Due to the positioning of Isaac's body in an elevated position with his feet lower than his head, he came to the room heavily sedated. Isaac's was on TPN liquid nutrition and arousing him to eat was not a concern. Rather, monitoring the swelling of the brain and his vital signs became of paramount importance. As day became night, Dr. Klimo became concerned as very little spinal fluid was draining into the surgical bag placed on the side of the bed.

On the second night, Dacia called me at midnight as Isaac's condition had taken a turn for the worse. Quickly I got dressed and made my way to the hospital. I could tell by her strained voice Isaac's life was hanging in the balance. Dr. Klimo had been called in the middle of the night as emergency surgery became necessary. When the surgeon arrived, Isaac's vital signs were dropping as the massively enflamed brain could no longer sustain the body's ability to control heart rate and blood pressure. As Isaac left the room, I wondered if we would ever see him alive again. I was unable to pull back my thoughts from what could possibly be an end of Isaac's young life. As the hours passed, I could only hope there would be answers when Dr. Klimo returned. The second operation would last three hours. I distinctly remember the surgeon's painful words when he returned to our room, "Isaac is in recovery and stable, but the operation was not successful. I have done everything medically I know to do but the swelling of his brain will not come down." A fellow from the surgery team told us later Dr. Klimo would be holding a conference call with his colleagues from around the United States. He reiterated the best surgeons in the world would be discussing Isaac's case.

As darkness fell, Dacia and I remember staring at the large video board in the PICU which displayed Isaac's vital signs. He had not been awake for three days. We became fixated on what we felt kept him alive – his will to survive. I told Dacia it would be best if she went back to our apartment to get some rest. We had a long hospital stay ahead of us. As I drifted off into a restless sleep, I was suddenly awaked by the sound of alarm bells going off in the room. I looked up to blue lights flashing in the hall. As I glanced at the clock, I could only conclude death had come calling at 3:00 AM. In fear, I saw Isaac's vital signs dropping to a dangerously low level. Oxygen and heart rate were on the verge of collapse. Once again, there came over Isaac a motionless tranquility as if he were going to pass from this life to the next. However, one of the fellows from the surgeon's team arrived and opened a valve to manually pull fluid off Isaac's brain. Roughly two minutes later Isaac's vital signs began to slowly recover. Due to Isaac being in a drug induced coma there was no way to communicate with him and assess his neurological signs. In addition to cancer, there existed a larger unresolved persistent problem threatening Isaac's life - swelling on his brain.

We are Behind the Eight Ball

T he next morning Dr. Klimo arrived after having a long conference call with his colleagues from around the United States. He ordered the nurses to place Isaac in a trans-limber position with his head lower than his feet. Previously, the team was trying to use the force of gravity to reduce swelling by elevating his head. Dr. Klimo believed Isaac had an extremely rare condition known as *hydrocephalus,* a condition of fluid buildup around the brain. The team believed this was brought about due to Isaac having low brain pressure. To reduce swelling the doctors wanted spinal fluid to rush to the head and thus increase the pressure to force it out from around the brain.

For the first time in six days, the surgical bag hanging on the side of the bed began to fill with fluid. Isaac was still in a drug induced coma, but his vital signs were strong. Early in the afternoon Isaac was taken back for an MRI scan to confirm the diagnosis and evaluate the need for an additional surgery. The doctors determined the brain shunt which had been placed during surgery in Tulsa was the wrong device. The shunt was designed to drain excess spinal fluid to the stomach using a small tube. However, the scan revealed the need to reopen an original hole in the back of the brain to allow the normal absorption of spinal fluid into the body. Due to the risk of infection from the line coming out of Isaac's head, surgery was of utmost importance. However, Isaac was a cancer patient, and something had gone wrong with the surgical implanted double Hickman lines in his chest. The operation was placed on hold.

The next morning Dr. Klimo was the bearer of bad news. A staph infection had developed in Isaac's bloodstream because of the Hickman lines. The infected blood cultures had to clear before the operation could commence. Dr. Klimo was direct regarding Isaac's prognosis, "If the infected blood cultures do not start to clear by tomorrow afternoon, call your family and friends. They must get here before the weekend if they want to see Isaac alive before he passes. This will all be over by Sunday night, unless the new antibiotics are successful. I'm truly sorry but we are behind the eight ball right now."

Sitting in the beautiful garden at St. Jude marking the burial site of its founder Danny Thomas, I remember hearing children walking outside. The sounds of their laughter and play were dreamlike as I pondered yet again the death of my oldest son. Isaac was so resilient; it was hard to fathom a staph infection would be his demise. I could not help but wonder how I would survive? How could I possibly tell Caleb he would be an only child? Contemplating returning home without him would bring back memories of an innocent life taken by the perils associated with cancer. Fighting back tears, I began to remember the life of Danny Thomas and his vision to build a hospital which would serve as a beacon of hope to the brokenhearted. Reflecting on his vision that "No child should die in the dawn of life," gave me strength during one of the most crucial times in my life.

In my brokenness and sorrow, I left the pavilion with a reaffirmed vow to never look back. I would not allow this crisis to define my battered life nor would I permit this catastrophe to ruin my family. Rather, I would chart a new course in life for better or worse. There would be no turning back as to finding the answer as to why this happened to Isaac. I would protect my family from the ravages of this disease and would try to leave it behind.

Waiting on the blood culture results the next morning would cause me to not sleep the night before. Isaac's life was now defined by the laboratory blood sample growing in the lab. I will never forget my restrained exhilaration when the doctor came by the next morning and said surgery had been scheduled for two o'clock in the afternoon. Yet again Isaac was not ready to give up his soul – the battle against cancer would go on.

H.O.P.E.
Hold On, Pain Ends

D r. Klimo was successfully able to surgically reopen the hole in the back of Isaac's brain to allow for the natural flow of excess spinal fluid to be absorbed into the body. Scar tissue had formed over the area which was the original reason for installing a nonprogrammable shunt six months prior in Tulsa. Recovery from brain surgery was quick as St. Jude was anxious to get Isaac back on their campus in preparation for the end of the clinical trial. Three days later we discharged back to St. Jude for the final round of chemotherapy.

The culmination of three previous chemo rounds and a sixteen-day detour due to the brain shunt failure made this procedure by far the most difficult. Not only did Isaac come into this cycle in a weakened state, but also in a wheelchair from being in bed for so long. After the second cycle of chemotherapy Isaac had been fitted for leg braces which he wore throughout the day. The braces were cast to prevent permanent damage from foot drop, which began occurring in his legs due to the chemo drug vincristine weakening the nerves in his legs. Isaac hated wearing the braces but the long-term prognosis for throwing them to the side was a wheelchair for life.

I remember dreading this final phase of the trial. We had checked into the hospital and were admitted to the Bone Marrow Transplant *(BMT)* floor. I vividly remember the onset of a fever only hours after the first chemotherapy drugs were administered through an IV drip. Isaac's feeble body began shaking violently and his teeth chattered as his body temperature rose to one hundred six degrees. The nausea and diarrhea came in unrelenting waves. At one point, I glanced at his chart only to notice he was taking thirty-five different medications. Numerous antibiotics were given as Isaac's body had no ability to fight off infection on its own. He was also taking medications for blood pressure, heart rhythm, kidney function, bladder spasms and anti-nausea to name just a few. The chemotherapy drugs had quickly stripped away any resemblance of an immune system, so precautions had to be taken when both entering the floor and room. Hand washing, gowns, masks and gloves were required on every visit as were restrictions on who could see him.

Once again, I gave witness to Isaac's body being forced to the verge of major organ failure and death. However, the excellent work of St. Jude in the field of stem cell therapy gave us courage our son would be one of the eighty-three percent who would survive. Isaac would remain in the hospital for nineteen days during this final cycle of chemotherapy. In between the critical areas came visits from other professionals. One of which was with our physical therapist Janet. It was on a day towards the end of our hospital stay when I finally began to see meaning in the word H.O.P.E. – **Hold On, Pain Ends.**

Prison Rules

The final round of chemotherapy was difficult in more than one way. Isaac had been in a bed for so long, he was weak and found walking very difficult. The nursing staff were closely monitoring a bed sore which had developed on his right side - thus he was not eager to participate in physical therapy. Begrudgingly, he put on his gown, mask and gloves as he went to the PT room. I came along too as I felt I might be able to motivate him to participate in the session. Due to being on the bone marrow transplant floor, I wore the same medical protective clothing as Isaac.

Today, our physical therapist Janet said we would try something new. She went into a nearby adjacent room and came out with some hockey sticks. Gently, she placed the puck on the floor and explained the basic rules. Lightly push the puck back and forth using your arms in the process. Isaac's first attempt at hitting the puck suggested his displeasure with participating. I hit it back only to see him stagger and refuse to chase it down. Realizing he might need some motivation, I called out, "Hey Isaac, how about we play by prison rules?" Isaac responded, "Are you serious?" At this point, I smashed the puck at the back wall and Isaac yelled, "Ok dad, you're on." Isaac ran after the puck and hit it as hard as he could right at me. Janet in bewilderment yelled, "Boys, what are prison rules?" Isaac's answer brought a smile and laugh I had not seen in a long time, "It means there are no rules!"

We would laugh about this therapy session for years to come. Each time on our quarterly visit to Memphis, we had a physical therapy consult on our schedule. All Janet could do was shake her head and say, "Prison rules, never in my life has anyone played a game like this during physical therapy."

In some respects, it was a turning point in this long battle with cancer. At the time, Isaac was bound to a wheelchair due to weakened muscles in his legs. Walking required the use of leg braces fitted to his feet. He would often cry and refuse to do the therapy stretches which were required two times a day. From this point forward we would joke about doing them by prison rules. In a small way, no rules brought about a desire to get well and end the unrelenting pain of cancer.

NED

The leaves in early November began to change colors and the end of the final chemotherapy cycle had finally arrived. During the hospital discharge process, a long and laborious task, something special happened which we did not expect. The door swung open and a group of nurses assembled in our room. One threw a can of confetti in the air and another said, "Isaac, we are here to celebrate your *No Mo Chemo Party!*" St. Jude has a customary celebration to mark the momentous day. One brought in a small gift and another a piece of cake. Isaac had not eaten any food in nearly seven months, so I took it upon myself to take care of it for him. Isaac bashfully said very little, but a distinctive smile appeared on the one side of his mouth which would move. The festive atmosphere would be tempered by news which would complicate his release from the bone marrow transplant floor – a strong intestinal infection would require Isaac be placed in isolation. Isaac would spend nearly four days in the apartment set apart from the hospital floors. His intestinal infection was highly contagious. We had to carefully bathe and care for his needs while protecting ourselves. Looming on the horizon was Christmas, and an opportunity to go home. However, it would be nearly six weeks before we headed home to the Sooner State.

We quickly came to realize our journey to Oklahoma would be a complicated maze of appointments with specialists, to gain clearance in completing the clinical trial. Isaac had numerous appointments with neuro-surgery, neurology, speech, physical therapy and oncology. Each specialty would evaluate Isaac's progress and monitor his recovery as it related to their research on his disease. Our oncologist Dr. Giles Robinson's words would unshackle a torment of fear when I heard him say, "Isaac is NED!" Somewhat puzzled and in quick fashion, I asked what it meant. This three-letter acronym would be the most defining declaration in Isaac's long journey with cancer. Dr. Giles said, "It means there is no evidence of disease. We call it NED for short." This apparent good news however, came with a sacrificial warning as the doctor went on to say, "Statistically within your clinical trial there is a very small chance the disease will reoccur within two years. There are no second chances, no one has ever lived from a relapse of this type of cancer."

In subsequent years when Isaac underwent an MRI, I would feel my stomach churn and my thoughts chained to the hope we would hear the word "NED," from the oncologist. NED is for every cancer survivor the anticipation life will be free of the affliction and suffering cancer treatment brings. For Isaac, NED became the aspiration to reclaim the life he once knew as an athlete, student and teenager.

However, on the horizon was one more surgery to correct the facial paralysis on the left side of his face. Cancer treatment had come to a close, however a crusade to rid Isaac's body of the devastation the treatments had left behind, would begin soon.

Cross Facial Nerve Surgery

Once again, we found ourselves at Le Bonheur Children's Hospital. The surgery prep area was customarily cold just like the weather outside. It was December 13, 2011 and the thought of actually being home at Christmas was a prize, worth praying the operation went well. Our neurosurgeon today was a kind and spirited man named Dr. Michael Muhlbauer. I found his bedside manner to be cheerful and actually quite funny. He put us at ease when he told Isaac his incision would go from his head to his toes but not to worry, he had done this more times than he could count. We laughed but quizzically Isaac said, "Are you serious doc?"

The surgeon explained the seventh cranial nerve which provides movement to the left side of the face was damaged during a tumor resection surgery last spring. The seventh cranial nerve was attached to the spinal cord in the same area in which the massive tumor was removed last March. Surgery today would be twofold, move the twelfth nerve of the tongue to work the left side of the face, and reroute a nerve from the neck to work the left side of the tongue in Isaac's mouth. The results would not be immediate as it takes a minimum of 6 months for the nerves to heal and regenerate movement on the left side of the face. Further, intense speech therapy would be required in the coming months as new patterns of swallowing would need to be taught.

Prior to surgery, Isaac's bell's palsy had been rated as a 6/6 on the facial nerve grading system. The surgeon told us he had only two percent functioning on the left side of his face. If successful, the operation today would restore some movement and move the marker to a 3/6. Facial symmetry would be normal in a resting position but closure of the eyelid and movement in the forehead would still be lost. In short, the smile would still be distorted but a noticeable "droop," in facial posture would be removed.

Dr. Muhlbauer told us it would take several hours to complete the surgery. His nurse said it better when she remarked, "Doctors don't know how to tell time but I will call you every hour and give an update." Unlike the cancer related operations, this was considered an elective surgery. I had a different feeling in the waiting room today. I began to contemplate how this might help Isaac as he returned to a normal world with the frailties and blemishes cancer treatment had left behind. My aspiration now was to provide Isaac with the protective bubble he would need to return to school and ultimately succeed as a young man in life. In more ways than one, I wanted this surgery to restore his ability to feel secure in a cruel world which would stare at his wounds and look at him as if he were a damaged child. The thought of being home for Christmas as a family would bring a smile to my face as did Dr. Muhlbauer walking into the waiting room.

Dr. Muhlbauer told us Isaac did fine during the five-hour operation. The surgeon had to literally make a six-inch incision from the ear to the base of the chin to move the nerves. He considered the operation successful but reiterated the need for speech therapy as chewing and swallowing food would be an immediate concern. Further, as the nerves begin to regenerate movements, a skilled therapist would be required to help Isaac learn new speech patterns.

If all went as planned, Isaac would be discharged within five days. However, he would still need to see an eye surgeon, and his neuro-oncologist before his final release from St. Jude. Christmas, being only a few days away, required a carefully planned maze of appointments in which everything had to go just right.

Homecoming

As we pulled out of the St. Jude parking lot, I felt an uneasiness and apprehensive spirit overcome me. For the first time since arriving in Memphis almost ten months ago, we were coming home as a family of three. The St. Jude doctors and medical professionals we came to trust and rely upon would now be four hundred miles away. Feeling as if we were setting off into an uncharted world, I began to ponder the future ahead of us. Isaac had survived the perils of cancer treatment, but he was bruised and weak from surgery. His fragile emotions would be tested by the return to a world unaware of what he had overcome. Further, Christmas was only three days away and in most years our home would be decorated with lights along with a Christmas tree. Due to a mid-December surgery and the hectic pace of packing to return home, we had not even had the time to go Christmas shopping for the boys. In a feeling of utter bewilderment and panic, I thought of ways to tell the boys Christmas presents would be delayed this year.

We were aware two close friends, Lisa Clark and Janet Pitts secretly put together an effort to bring Christmas joy and traditions to the Walsh family. Janet had worked with her lady's sorority group to purchase food for the pantry and stock the refrigerator. In all fairness, it was a surprise to the boys but be ensured the food provided was a favorite of Isaac and Caleb *(we sent a list beforehand)*. Lisa Clark, who worked as a PE teacher for me and had Isaac in class, arranged for the Christmas tree to be put up in our back room complete with decorations and ornaments. There were Christmas lights hanging on the trees in our front yard. As we pulled into the driveway approximately eighty people encompassing our friends, family, church members and neighbors had gathered to welcome us home. Some held signs of encouragement while others cheerfully waved. A large banner with the words *Welcome Home Isaac* with OKC Thunder basketball logo hung prominently as if this were staking out the home of a Hollywood celebrity. As Isaac stepped out of the car, a sudden scream of *"Welcome home,"* reverberated throughout the neighborhood. I noticed near the front porch our younger son Caleb, he came running to greet us and was smiling. I remember distinctly his words to his older brother Isaac, "There are presents under the tree."

In every person's life there comes a time when one is at loss for words to express their gratitude and thanks. Words are not enough to express the emotions and love I felt on this cold December night. It would be more than a homecoming for one child who survived the ravages of cancer. Rather, it was a celebration of life reminding us all of the steadfast devotion of friends and family. As I went to bed later, I was reminded of what I had seen on many t-shirts and banners during the St. Jude Marathon we had watched only two weeks ago, "No one fights alone." Despite our friends and family being four hundred miles away they were with us, all the time.

Part IV
Survivorship Years

Cross Facial Nerve Graft Surgery

A lthough Isaac had been discharged from St. Jude, we had joined a clinical trial which required a commitment to return to Memphis for further study. Each time there would be a four-day battery of tests and exams to study the side effects of the cancer drugs which had been given experimentally. Usually before each trip to Memphis, I would feel my anxiety build as we had met several parents along our journey who buried their son or daughter, as a result of battling this disease. However, as the years began to pass so too did my fear of a relapse of cancer. Plaguing Isaac as he entered his high school years was his malformed face. Despite having completed years of intense speech therapy there was little movement on the left side of the face. This would change when we met St. Jude plastic surgeon Dr. Robert Wallace.

Dr. Wallace's proposed surgery would be two-fold. First, nerves on the outer side of the legs working the pinky toes would be removed and grafted to the face. The surgeon would open the working side of the face (*right*) and connect the nerve tissues removed from the legs. In the final part of the first operation, he would tunnel them under the nose, mouth and chin to provide movements to the paralyzed side.

A second operation commonly known as the "smile," surgery would involve grafting muscle from his thigh to the paralyzed side of the face. This complicated procedure had been done hundreds of time by Dr. Wallace and he was among a handful of surgeons who had the skills to perform this type of microsurgery. Further, the operation involved connecting muscle fibers, suturing together blood vessels and constantly monitoring for blood clots which could cause the entire surgery to fail. The overall success rate for this surgery was ninety-five percent.

In some ways, I was reluctant to proceed with this type of surgery. As I let my mind wander back to the cancer related procedures just three years ago, a raw set of emotions began to set in - I pondered what could possibly go wrong. The thought of losing him over an elective procedure was something I didn't know if I could ever heal from. What if his face was worse after the procedure? Dr. Wallace's compassionate bedside manner, and Isaac's insistence on wanting to wipe away a leftover image from his battle with the disease won me over.

Dr. Wallace scheduled the surgery to begin on July 24, 2014 and unlike many cancer related operations this one would be completed at St. Jude. The procedure lasted eight hours, with the nurse calling us on the top of the hour with updates from the operating room. We met with the surgeon in the late afternoon and he told us Isaac had forty-five stitches in each of his legs and sixty on his face. A large six-inch incision from the base of the ear to the chin had caused considerable swelling on his face. It would be nine months before the nerves would completely heal, and the second phase of transplanting muscle could begin.

Facial Reanimation *"Smile"* Surgery

S omewhat naive, I never really asked about the full scope of the facial reanimation surgery in terms of days in the hospital and the immediate outlook following the operation. However, in a meeting with Dr. Wallace a week prior to surgery in his east Memphis office, I began to have second thoughts on proceeding with the muscle transplant. The average stay in the hospital for this type of operation was four days but could be much longer if complications arose. Moreover, this was not a life or death event where surgery had to be done to eradicate cancer from the body. Rather, this was an elective surgery we chose to do on our own. St. Jude would pay all surgery, hospital and doctor fees as they looked at this as a cancer related operation for children left with a deformed face. For many a drooping face caused speech and swallowing issues. If successful, Isaac's smile and facial function on the left side of his face would be almost ninety percent back to normal. In a small way, it would erase the tarnished picture he saw of himself each time he looked into a mirror.

The second stage began nine months after the nerve graft procedure in April 2015. Due to the complexity of the procedure, the operation was being done at nearby Le Bonheur Children's Hospital. In addition, Dr. Wallace had a team of surgeons assisting him as he expected the operation to last a minimum of sixteen hours. Once again, I found myself sitting in a hospital waiting room eager for the phone to ring on the top of every hour, informing us of how surgery was progressing. The crushing weight of cancer was gone, but the quest to help Isaac reclaim a part of his life filled my mind with thoughts of how this might change his outlook on life. Could it really be possible this surgery would restore the confidence and self-assurance his personality afforded him prior to cancer? My thoughts were transfixed on a possibly new reality this surgery could bring, a life set free from the scars of cancer. As day faded into night, Dr. Wallace appeared around eight o'clock in the evening to brief us on the status of the operation.

Surgery was still ongoing and likely would be finished around midnight. Isaac would be moved to an ICU room due to the complications of monitoring both a wound on his inner thigh and an open flap on his face where the transplanted muscle was placed. Trained nurses with doppler sonar devices would monitor blood flow every thirty minutes to assess blood clotting. Further, Isaac would be placed in a drug induced coma in a paralyzed state and on a ventilator for a minimum of three days to prevent any type of movement which might rip apart the micro-sutured blood vessels and muscle fibers.

I realized our stay in the hospital would go beyond the normal four days when Isaac's veins began clotting, and emergency surgery became necessary to clear the blockage. The surgeon would come by our room four hours later and tell us the clot was successfully removed, but there was serious concern due to swelling on both the face and in the legs. Blood loss at times had been severe, as at one point he was losing two liters every four hours, and they couldn't wake him to assess his neurological signs. This would be too risky according to the surgeon as any slight movement could easily split apart the muscle fibers and ruin the transplanted veins. The possibility of an infection in his lungs due to a prolonged time spent on a ventilator was now a pressing concern. At the time, I found myself at a crossroads thinking if we pursued on with more surgery, this might cost Isaac his life, let alone the long sought after smile the operation itself sought to restore.

It was Friday night and as is customary the hospital emergency room began to get busy. The sound of the Life

Flight helicopter reminded me of the trauma center situated in another wing of the hospital. Around midnight, our alert nurse began to notice a change in the doppler patterns. Isaac was losing excessive amounts of blood - the plastic surgeon was immediately called. For the first time since we had completed our cancer treatment protocol at St. Jude, I began to worry as they took him away to surgery. I sensed there would be no second chances on clearing the clot and waiting a few more days to close the open flap. Rather, due to the persistence of continual clotting and the risk of an infection in his lungs, this had become a critical decision. I remember telling the surgeon to do whatever needs to be done to save his life.

Four hours later, the surgeon came humbly back to our room and told us the transplanted muscle had to be pulled and face sutured closed. Isaac would not lose any previously restored facial functioning and x-rays of his chest showed no infection in his lungs. In addition, he would be handing over the process of awakening Isaac from a drug induced coma to a team of ICU doctors, who would monitor his neurological signs as the paralytic drugs were weaned off. He would stop by daily and talk with us later about other options.

Dr. Wallace's dejected face spoke volumes of how badly he wanted this surgery to be successful for Isaac. He had formed a special bond with him and wanted to restore part of the life Isaac once knew. Dr. Wallace would tell us a year later, their study revealed clotting under the transplanted muscle had caused the ultimate end of the procedure. Knowing the anatomy of Isaac's face and his response to the first unsuccessful attempt at surgery, he felt a second try would be successful.

Isaac had reserved emotions about trying surgery again. In reality, his badly bruised face took months to heal. In some ways, he came to accept his face would never be normal again.

In retrospect, I wonder if I pushed him to reconsider his options to have surgery. Isaac was eighteen years old at the time, it would be his decision alone. Much like most teens, insurance and the factor of who will pay for this type of elective surgery doesn't seem to show up on their radar. Knowing the window of St. Jude paying for the procedure and Dr. Wallace's retirement one day, Isaac signed the consent papers to move forward with another attempt at facial reanimation. Due to an allergic reaction to a drug given at the start of surgery, Isaac once again came to the precipice of death. Unlike three precious times, Isaac actually died at the start of the operation and had to be revived.

"We Lost Him"

T he second attempt at facial reanimation surgery had been similar to the first. The drug induced coma, ventilator, emergency surgery to clear common clots and blood transfusions were all something we came to expect. Due to the previous failed attempt, a larger team of surgeons was brought in to complete the twenty-five-hour operation. However, it was on day eleven when a routine trip to the operating room reminded me life is fragile and can turn on the drop of a dime.

The door to the consult room opened as both Dr. Wallace and his assistant appeared in their surgical gear. I could tell by their shaken appearance something had gone seriously wrong. We were told the operation would last approximately one hour but it had stretched to seven and a half. I began to intensely study Dr. Wallace's facial expression. I became instantly seized with fear when I saw a tear in his eye. In a suspended state of panic and alarm, I distinctly remember only the first three words Dr. Wallace spoke when he said, "We lost him." Isaac was given a common anti-clotting drug routinely administered through an IV drip to stop severe blood loss at the start of surgery. Instantly, despite having only received a quarter teaspoon of the drug, his body began to shake and swelling appeared in his face. His airway became cut off and all breathing stopped. A massive anaphylactic shock occurred and the code blue alarms began to go off. A team of resuscitation doctors and nurses rushed into the room in a successful effort to revive him. The surgeon would later relay if Isaac had not been prepped for surgery with a ventilator down his trachea, he would have passed within thirty seconds.

It would take nearly five hours for Isaac to be stabilized for the surgery to continue. The clot was successfully removed but the presence of more blockages persisted overnight. Isaac's doctor stayed by his side as darkness fell on the hospital. In a remarkable and reverent show of compassion, the surgeon dressed his wounds and oversaw the eighteen blood transfusions given overnight. As the sun came across the horizon, I could only try to push the previous night out of my memory. Not since we were told Isaac had very little chance to survive the initial cancer resection surgery nearly seven years ago, did I feel so helpless and vulnerable to the fear of losing him. Notwithstanding, my raw emotions became more apparent when Isaac was taken back for surgery again around noon the next day. My only words to the plastic surgeon as I signed the surgery consent papers were, "Please don't let him die."

Isaac would come back two hours later with the muscle graft removed and his face stitched closed. Dr. Wallace's words would remind me the victory over cancer could not be comprised by a surgery to restore a smile when he said, "I removed the transplanted muscle and closed up his face. I could not in my best medical judgement risk losing him again. I'm sorry but there will be no more surgery to restore his smile."

Much like before, the process of awakening Isaac from a prolonged drug induced coma would come over the entirety of the next week. In my despair and sorrow, I began to contemplate how to tell him it was over, his smile could never be restored. More so, I began to worry how he would react again to a severely bruised face which bore no hope to a future of being normal again.

Isaac would gradually accept one of the permanent scars of cancer would be an imperfect smile. He has learned how to chew food, compensate for speech and maintain facial symmetry in a resting position. In some ways, his smile has become a trademark expression which he does not hide. For me, it's a reminder of a child who in the face of extreme adversity never gave up. More so, it was through the delicate hands of the medical professionals at St. Jude I can still see his smile today. Maybe one day we all will look at others through an unfiltered set of eyes, where a crooked smile is considered normal as we express our joy in life.

A Graduation Speech to the St. Jude Board of Directors

Numerous times throughout our stay in Memphis I spoke to various corporate groups about our family's journey with cancer. One such group was the St. Jude Board of Directors and Governors. This large body which oversees, the ALSAC Division of St. Jude welcomed me twice over the course of nine years. One such time was in May 2011 during Isaac's treatment. I was privileged to speak again on June 25, 2016 only one month after Isaac graduated from high school. The excerpt of my speech is noted below...

"...When I came to you five years ago, my child Isaac was undergoing cancer treatment at St. Jude. Today, I stand before you as a father of a five-year brain cancer survivor. Only one month ago, I watched my child graduate from high school. He was in the top twenty-five percent of his class and had received a full ride scholarship to a technical school to work on degree in internet security. As I sat in the stands on this historic night, I thought about where I'm standing right now – St. Jude. Due to the work of Danny Thomas and the vision he had that no child should die in the dawn of life, I was able to see my child make it to graduation day.

As I listened to the graduation honors, scholarships and athletic accomplishments read for the other students, I could only think of what Isaac had overcome to make it to this day. He did not have an athletic scholarship nor was he an All-State Scholar, rather he had been tested by the battle lines of cancer.

- *21 surgeries (Eight major brain surgeries and the longest lasting twenty-five hours)*
- *31 experimental treatments of radiation to the brain and spine*
- *4 experimental rounds of chemotherapy*
  - *Three FDA approved cancer fighting drugs doubled at the standard dose*
- *4 stem cell transplants to prevent major organ failure and ward off death*
- *125 blood transfusions*
- *Over one year spent in the hospital*
- *Three times Isaac lay on his deathbed as he would nearly succumb to the disease*
- *Number of medications Isaac takes long term as a result of cancer –1 (Over the counter vitamin D)*
- *Total cost of treatment thus far at St. Jude – $5 million dollars*
- *What our insurance company has paid - $2 million dollars*
- *The amount St. Jude has asked us to pay on an unpaid medical bill of $3 million dollars – Absolutely nothing (zero)*

As Isaac took his diploma and walked off the stage, tears began to fill my eyes. I thought this day would never come. Further, had it not been for the medical professionals and commitment of your Board to fund lifesaving cancer research, I would not be here today. Rather, I would be in a cemetery staring at a gravestone mourning the loss of a child whose life ended nearly five years ago. My son is alive today because of your faithful commitment to the values *which make St. Jude a beacon of hope for those who are lost in the whirlwinds of cancer.*

Words cannot express the gratitude I feel as your leadership has saved my family from financial ruin. We never had to choose between saving our child or selling our house – all because of you.

There are many who walk through the doors of this great hospital hoping to find a miracle to save their child's life. They come from all over the world, some are poor and speak a different language, but they are all welcomed here. Your group leads an extraordinary organization which I will forever be in their debt. I'm forever grateful..."

Tom Walsh
June 25, 2016

Caleb Walsh, Brother and Best Friend
Survivorship Years

I awoke early to the sound of laughter and playful screaming outside. It was summer and the sun was just coming above the horizon. At the time, our kids were not yet school age. Immediately, I became concerned when a quick peek in the boy's bedroom revealed there was no one there. Running to the backyard, I found both boys stripped of their clothes sliding on a wet trampoline. The family dog had joined in the fun too. The boys had hoisted him up onto the trampoline and were diving on top of him. It was the picture-perfect scene of two little boys enjoying man's best friend.

Early memories of childhood would remind Caleb of happier times. He recalled playing football in the front yard with his brother Isaac when he was nine years old. The cool crisp air along with the red and gold leaves etched a memory of a time when life was normal and void of pain. A time before tragedy struck – before his older brother would be diagnosed with brain cancer. Before life would never be the same.

Caleb would discuss with me, nine years after Isaac's diagnosis the agony of watching his older brother battle cancer - when the CT scan revealed the massive brain tumor. Caleb recalled, "I remember you telling me Isaac might not make it." He described the pain of watching his older brother return to the school hallways where he was once regarded as a little league all-star. Fighting back tears Caleb said, "It was hard for me to watch someone who was so talented athletically suffer so much." For months Caleb would watch as his older brother awkwardly and in an uncoordinated fashion walk between classes. Caleb became emotional when he reflected back to this painful time as he said, "I wanted Isaac to have his life back. I wish it had happened to me."

Caleb began to mature at a young age. His role became protector and guardian against the cruel stares which followed Isaac everywhere he went. As Isaac returned to the routines and schedule of a typical teen, his younger brother realized he would need a buddy. Caleb quickly became the more social of our two children. He began to include Isaac in his inner circle of friends and invited him to the activities he attended. Caleb was more than a brother to Isaac; he was also his best friend.

Caleb would follow in his brother's footsteps by attending a vocational school after graduation from high school. He earned a HVAC certificate and was hired by a large Tulsa firm specializing in commercial heat and air even before he completed school. Although it was difficult, Caleb would work an eight-hour day and later attend a four-hour class at night to complete his HVAC certification. As many in the HVAC industry do, he works long hours in the heat of summer.

As Caleb ponders his future, he wants to travel the world and meet new people. He often reflects on how this tragedy has changed his life. Tattooed on Caleb's left bicep are four letters – *MMXI* which are the Roman numerals for the year 2011. When I asked Caleb what it means to him, he answered in a profound manner by saying, "It was the year Isaac beat cancer, it made me realize nothing is impossible."

Memories of My Darkest Hour
By Dacia Walsh
(Edited by Tom Walsh)

Tom: Looking back what were the signs and symptoms which led you to believe Isaac was gravely ill?

Dacia: I knew something was seriously wrong. Isaac had been having severe headaches and was holding his head sideways like he had a muscle strain. He refused to eat and had lost a lot of weight. We had taken him to our family doctor who had run every test one could imagine. In all, Isaac had been to an optometrist, physical therapist, chiropractor, and we even took him to the emergency room only to be told he was dehydrated.

Tom: What do you remember about the day he was diagnosed with cancer?

Dacia: I remember when we were shown the CT scan and told Isaac had a tumor the size of a softball on his brainstem. Everything was moving quickly. I remember being told Isaac had cancer. I had lost my mom and my mother-in-law to cancer and now my son had it. I recall not being able to breathe, I didn't know what to say or think. These are times when you find out just how strong you are. I won't lie, I questioned why this was happening, but I also decided to not give up on my faith. Instead, I dedicated Isaac to God and thought His will be done whatever happens.

Tom: How hard was it for you to leave Tulsa to get Isaac the treatment he needed?

Dacia: *Isaac went through a series of surgeries at St. Francis, two of which were very critical and the danger of losing him was high. We had a decision to make about whether we would stay in Tulsa or go four hundred miles away to St. Jude Children's Research Hospital for treatment. This ended up being a "no brainer" decision as the success rate for this type of cancer was much higher at St. Jude. I was torn about going so far away because we had our younger son Caleb to consider as well.*

Tom: We received tremendous support from the people we knew back home. What would you like to say to the many people who expressed empathy and compassion towards our family?

Dacia: *The outpouring of love and support we received from our friends, family, church, and our community is something I will be forever grateful for. The monetary donations, food baskets and gift cards were all generous tokens of how much people cared. We even had neighbors who watched our house and mowed our lawn. There were also many people who invested their time in Caleb to make the transition easier for him. Lastly, the sick leave donations from the employees of Sapulpa Public Schools was overwhelming. As we headed off to Memphis, it was reassuring to know we had such a strong and loving support system in place. However, a part of my heart was left in Sapulpa, as we could not bring Caleb with us.*

Tom: What did you feel inside the day we arrived at St. Jude?

Dacia: *I had a mix of emotions. I will never forget the first time we walked through the doors of the hospital. We were met with bald headed kids being pulled in wagons, children pulling IV stands and some kids with prosthetic limbs. It stood out to me*

*when Isaac said, "It is not fair all these kids are sick."
Immediately, I thought to myself Isaac will soon be one of these
kids. I knew in a short amount of time; we would become part
of the St. Jude family.*

Tom: What stood out the most to you about St. Jude?

*Dacia: The place was not like your typical hospital. As you
walk through the hallways, you are immediately drawn to the
artwork, which is all completed by the children at St. Jude. The
emphasis being on what each child is going through with their
cancer. There are play areas and special "teen rooms" for the
older kids. Isaac liked the teen room, because mom and dad
were not allowed in. Unlike your typical hospital, the only
treatment ongoing at St. Jude is cancer. We met some
incredible families who became lifelong friends as their
struggle was the same as ours.*

Tom: St. Jude is a hospital unlike any other. Did you feel like
you made the right decision in going there?

*Dacia: Learning early on that we were not going to be billed
for anything while we were at St. Jude made me feel a little
more at ease. Our focus could be on getting Isaac well no
matter what the cost. We had a long road ahead of us with his
treatment. I had a sense of hope being here. The doctors in
charge of Isaac's case were the best in the world. They were
dedicated to finding a cure for cancer and making kids well. I
also found it interesting some of the staff at St. Jude had
previously been a patient at St. Jude when they were young. I
was comforted knowing my son was in the hands of people who
were truly passionate about their work.*

Tom: As you reflect back to Isaac's treatment, were there times when you thought this could be the end?

Dacia: The journey at St. Jude was long and tedious at times, but the end result was a miracle. Isaac endured twenty-one surgeries, thirty-one low grade radiation treatments and four experimental rounds of chemotherapy combined with stem cell therapy. There were many times we almost lost him, but he came through every time. I can remember standing next to his hospital bed and praying, "God please don't take him away from me, let him live." The strength, endurance, and the will to fight this horrible disease was self-evident in Isaac and is something that I drew from to get through the ordeal. Isaac is a fighter and I am happy to say he once was an employee at St. Jude. Survivorship has a whole new meaning for me now after losing my mom, mother-in-law, and almost my son to this horrible disease.

Tom: What was it like to finally come home and be reunited as a family again?

Dacia: *I often wondered what life was going to be like when we got back home to Sapulpa. During our time at St. Jude, we took turns going home to spend time with Caleb. I can remember a couple of times, one being around the time of my birthday I surprised Caleb with a visit. Those were special times and I cherished every one of them. Perspective is different for me now. I realize the God given gift of family and how precious it really is. I remember returning home just before Christmas and wondering what it was going to be like. Coming home to a fully decorated house, a pantry full of food, and many people lining my driveway was a blessing.*

Tom: It's often said a person adjusts to a new normal in their life after coming home. Would it be true for you as well?

Dacia: Isaac and Caleb settled in to a somewhat different normal. They couldn't play rough like they used to before Isaac had cancer. Although, it did not stop them, it was just at a different degree. School was heavy on everyone's mind as well. We took it slow, half days at first. Isaac would get very tired by the afternoon and emotional too. It would soon become apparent that we were not in the safety of St. Jude where Isaac looked like the other kids. For Isaac, he was back in the cruel setting of high school where kids would look at him funny and sneer because he had big scars on his head. My heart was broken the day I saw a group of girls doing this to him. The most difficult part of coming home was fitting back into a world unaware of what we had been through. The struggle was real, but Isaac accomplished it. He graduated high school and went on to receive a degree in Network Security Administration. Caleb also graduated from high school and received an associate degree in HVAC as a heat and air specialist.

Tom: Final thoughts?

Dacia: Our family has suffered a great deal. However, I believe we have become stronger for it. Through our faith in God and the support we had, the cancer battle has been won. We are not promised tomorrow, so I vow to live each day to the fullest in love and kindness toward one another.

I would like to close with words from a picture hanging in our home...

Thomas M. Walsh

What Cancer Can't Do

It can't prevent love
It can't conquer the spirit
It can't silence courage
It can't take away memories
It can't weaken faith
It can't defeat hope

My Journey to a Place of Hope and Healing
By Tom Walsh

I often tell people when a child suffers from a catastrophic illness such as cancer, the entire family is thrust into a state of upheaval and turmoil. For some, this cataclysmic event ends in a bitter divorce and leaves its mark by a trail of financial hardships and lifelong addictions. Realizing the quest to find the answer to the question as to why such a disease would strike a child can ruin a person's life. The anger and bitterness will lead to an empty obsession to understand one of life's unforeseen tragedies. In turn, this can cause despair, overwhelming pain and sorrow. I remember looking at Isaac in his hospital bed in Tulsa before he was wheeled away for surgery. The anguish I felt watching my child inches from the cliff of death is difficult to put into words. As for me, I made a vow on March 9, 2011 which would forever change my outlook on life and guide my thinking for years too come. It is listed below...

I will never allow myself to look back and wonder what could have been.

Returning to Oklahoma, I would never contemplate how much my life was changed due to cancer. Rather, our family would chart a new course appreciating each member as we enjoy our short time on earth together. I recalled on our second day back eating dinner at the table, how in times past I would chastise the boys when they would laugh and play during the dinner hour. Today would prove to be no different as Caleb looked at Isaac and started laughing for no reason. Isaac could only help by joining in this playful occasion. For me, it was a surreal moment as only a few months ago this day never seemed possible. This light-hearted time together soothed my bruised emotions and restored my belief our lives could be normal again.

The next morning, I walked into Isaac's room. I remember nudging him to the point he awoke, to make sure he had not passed away during the overnight hours. Gradually, I would come to accept the new normal cancer had brought to our lives. Vacation plans were tailored to what all members of the family were able to do. Ski vacations were replaced with trips to parks and ballgames, places where no family member would be defined by a disability, nor looked down on because they could not participate. Despite having no major medical problems, post cancer treatment, Isaac's life and transition would be difficult in a world which did not understand what he had been through. In some ways, the entire family adjusted to assisting and helping a recovering teenage cancer patient adapt to a normal world.

After a long break from working as a principal at an elementary school, I returned midyear after Isaac was released by St. Jude. My views as an administrator began to change as well. I would often tell my staff, the most important priority in your life needs to be your family. You will always have a job here at school but do not neglect your family. Long after your job is in the rear-view mirror, sitting beside you will be your children and spouse. Never let anything come between you and those whom you love the most.

On June 12, 2020 I retired at age fifty-three as a school administrator. My career would span three decades all within the same school district – Sapulpa Public Schools. It was also the year of the COVID-19 crisis and my final months would be marked by working from home or in a lonely office at school. As I walked away, I reminisced about the special role children played in my life. Their unbiased love, unselfish ambition to learn new things and the compassion they bestowed on me made it difficult to leave.

Shortly after my retirement, I contemplated the vow Danny Thomas made when he said, "No child should die in the dawn of life." For me, there is nothing more important than saving the life of a child. In my remaining years, I have passion to spread an awareness of pediatric cancer. Writing this book and sharing our intimate struggles is my first step in fulfilling my goal to be a part of the miracles occurring at St. Jude. I consider it to be the greatest honor of my life to share Isaac's cancer story. I often read over the intercom at school a quote from one of America's most beloved entertainers, it has become my rallying cry for the future.

All our dreams can come true if we have the courage to pursue them. – Walt Disney

Present Day
Summer 2020

Isaac's cancer treatments have been in our distant past for almost nine years now. Despite having been discharged from St. Jude back in December 2011, Isaac underwent numerous surgeries post cancer. His final surgery occurred in July 2019.

As of today, Isaac lives a relatively normal life with only routine cancer checkups. They are required annually as part of the St. Jude clinical trial we joined after he was diagnosed with cancer. Initially, due to brain seizure activity after a major surgery, Isaac had to be cleared by a neurologist in order to get an Oklahoma driver's license. However, Isaac has been seizure free for almost eight years now and this restriction has ended. As with most cancer related treatments, picking up the pieces of a broken life are almost as difficult as the treatment itself. As for Isaac, he attempted to find his place in the world by returning to the very hospital which saved his life.

Isaac graduated from a technical school in May 2016 and a few days later accepted a job in the IT department at St. Jude. I starkly remember the day we dropped him off at his garage apartment in an upscale area of Memphis near the campus of St. Jude. Isaac was excited to start his new life, but I was reluctant to let him go. Watching him wave goodbye as we drove away brought back painful memories of the early surgery in Tulsa where his prognosis was very grim. In the months which followed, I would monitor his movements on our *"Find My Friends,"* app in an effort to make sure something tragic did not happen to him. As time passed, so did my worry about Isaac living so far from home.

As Isaac started work at St. Jude, he realized the hospital is a multibillion-dollar corporation with over four thousand employees. His new coworkers had never met a St. Jude patient. Although working on the same campus where he once walked the halls as a cancer-stricken child, the business side of St. Jude was something Isaac had never seen before. He was reluctant to share his story, and in some ways attempted to dismiss this part of his past - the part which brought him so much pain. Isaac never connected with his peers in Memphis, something needed for him to flourish so far from home. The COVID-19 health crisis, and the quarantine work requirements, brought on a sense of despair and loneliness which prompted Isaac to look for a job in Tulsa, Oklahoma. Soon thereafter, Isaac accepted a job at the newly built Amazon Fulfillment Center near Tulsa International Airport in October 2020.

Our youngest son Caleb went to a technical school and graduated with a degree in HVAC. As is customary in the hotter climates in the southern United States, Caleb works long hours during the summer months. At the young age of twenty, Caleb left home and rented an apartment with a roommate in nearby Tulsa. He enjoys playing golf, riding a dirt bike and spending time with friends.

Caleb has grown up in the shadows of the attention bestowed upon Isaac. Reflecting back on this part of his life is difficult and a source of suffering. He has always been a person who demonstrated empathy towards others. Watching his older brother battle pediatric brain cancer has been very painful for Caleb to process. However, Caleb remains very close to his brother and enjoys his friendship.

As for Dacia and me, our lives resembled a scattered puzzle nine years ago. As parents of a pediatric cancer survivor, we have found not all the pieces fit together as they once did prior to Isaac having cancer. Despite having miraculously survived, Isaac has many limitations and we had to strive to find a balance of meeting his needs along with managing those of our family. Summer vacations were arranged around Isaac's cancer related appointments, and we alternated going to Memphis for his quarterly visits after returning home. In many respects, our lives revolved around meeting Isaac's needs and trying to provide equal time for his younger brother Caleb, who resembled a *"normal,"* healthy child.

Dacia retired from public education in the summer of 2019. Her career spanned two school districts primarily teaching fifth grade and small group reading. She currently works as a relationship banker at First United Bank in Sapulpa. Dacia is also a US Army military veteran who served stateside during the first Gulf War. Lastly, she enjoys spending time with family, reading, traveling and biking.

As for me, I walked away from education in the summer of 2020 to an uncertain future. Due to the COVID-19 pandemic my future plans to speak at corporate events and symposiums were placed on hold. In the interim, I have a normal exercise routine of biking and/or walking. In addition, there are a plethora of household chores which were neglected over the past twenty years which keep me busy. I also have plans to travel.

I would love to go visit the orphanage in El Salvador where I have served two previous times as a volunteer. Connecting with children who come from a troubled past brings me joy and peace. I once told the orphanage director; "A person cannot come to a place like this and not fall in love with those who are considered by many to be a *"damaged child."* My hope is one day the rest of my family will get a chance to meet these heroic kids. Just like Isaac survived cancer, an orphan child must pick up the pieces of their shattered life and make a new beginning. As I ponder my future in publishing, compiling and sharing the stories of an orphan child might be the next book I write.

Afterword
In My Own Words by Isaac Walsh
(Edited and Written by Tom Walsh)

A lmost nine years had passed since Isaac was diagnosed with cancer. For years, Isaac refused to talk about his intimate feelings as he coped with the disease. However, on a hot summer day in Memphis, Tennessee during the quarantine of the COVID-19 crisis, he finally opened up and talked about how he really felt.

Tom: You mentioned wanting to say something for this book. What do you want people to know?

Isaac: The hardest part of having cancer was not having cancer itself. During treatment, I always knew someone would always be there for me. It might be you, mom or a nurse – I was never alone. However, when I came home it was much different. Going back into the real world was the hardest for me. I knew that I was never going to be normal again but when I accepted it, I realized I would be better than normal. I would be a limited edition! Going back to the house where I grew up as a kid filled me with a lot of childhood memories. I was frustrated when I could not do many of those things as a result of cancer.

Tom: What were some of the activities you were not able to do?

Isaac: I was not able to ride a bike and I couldn't even shoot a basketball. I wasn't able to play football with my brother Caleb or even able to jump on the trampoline. It left me angry as other people had to do things for me. I had to adjust to a new way of living.

Tom: What was it like returning to school? Could you tell people stared at you?

Isaac: *Yeah, people still look at me every day. Back then, I was bald, and all the teenagers could see the large surgery scars on my head. The kids only stopped to say hi because they felt sorry for me. I don't know if anyone knew this but there were times when I wanted to die. I just didn't want to deal with it all. However, it was people such as my close friends, family and those who have been in my life which gave me hope. They are why I'm still here today.*

Tom: You came back into a world which did not understand what you had been through. It would have been easy for you to curl up and shut out the rest of the world. Were you upset about being forced to go back to school?

Isaac: *I hated school and did not want to go. I went to school with most of these kids for many years. I don't blame them for not understanding as when I came down with cancer everything changed. I felt like a new student in a familiar place. There were times when I felt the person who wrote this quote.*

> *"The bravest thing I ever did was continuing my life when I wanted to die." – Juliette Lewis*

Tom: If you could say anything to those people now. What would it be?

Isaac: *Many people will say since I had cancer that's who I am now. I don't think what they say is true, it's only a part of who I am.*

Tom: Did you find acceptance anywhere after coming home?

Isaac: *When I came back home, I hated school and didn't want to go. One thing I did want to do and enjoyed was going to my church youth group. I felt like this part of my life never changed. Before I came down with the disease, everyone in the youth group would say I was crazy, funny, and smart. When they got the news about me having cancer, they couldn't believe it. They came to the hospital to have Wednesday night class with me. When I couldn't be with them due to my illness, they had a handkerchief with my name written on it. They prayed over it every time they got together while I was away. Later Pastor Jon gave me the handkerchief. I still have it with me to this day. When I came back to the youth group after being away at St. Jude, everyone was so glad to see me. I was thrilled to be back for good. It's almost like everyone said, "He's back!"*

Tom: Going back to what you mentioned earlier, how did you overcome your attitude of wanting to die?

Isaac: *I never really thought seriously about ending my life. Rather, I had just hoped I would die and end it all. However, I realized having a bad attitude would affect everyone around me. Cancer hit me so fast and limited what I could do. I changed my attitude.*

Tom: You mentioned an influential movie which changed your attitude. Can you tell me more about it?

Isaac: *I saw the movie Facing the Giants (2006 film by Sherwood Pictures) and remember a scene where the coach has the star player death crawl with someone on his back across the field. The player asked the coach, you want me to go to the thirty-yard line? Then the coach said no I think you can go to the fifty. I want you to give me your absolute best. His coach then went onto to say he had to do it blindfolded so he wouldn't give up when he could go further. At the end, the coach took the blindfold off and said look up - you're in the endzone. The coach told him you are the most influential player on this team, if you walk around defeated so will they. God has gifted you with the ability of leadership so don't waste it. Your attitude affects everyone around you.*

Tom: People will often look at the six-inch scar on your head where the tumor was removed. What does this scar mean to you?

Isaac: *Although I'm not bald now, you can still see my scars from my twenty-one surgeries. I call my scars tattoos with better stories! So, when people stare at me, they are looking at the stories which tried to kill me.*

Tom: What does the saying, *"I had cancer, but it never had me,"* mean to you?

Isaac: *Cancer took my athletic ability, but it can never strip away my personality. Nor my love for life itself.*

Tom: What's next for you?

Isaac: *I want to get married and have kids. I want to own my own home and be financially set. However, first I want to get a* *good job to be able to provide for them. There is a poster which said it best called "Don't Skip Steps."*

Step # 1: Education   Step # 2: Career
Step # 3: Love   Step # 4: Marriage

Tom: What advice would you give to someone else your age who has cancer?

Isaac: I would like to tell those who have cancer going back into the real world will be the hardest thing you do. It would have been easy for me to shut the rest of the world out by doing drugs, drinking alcohol and curling up so no one could see me. However, you are the CEO of your life. You can't let cancer nor other people bring you down. You must own yourself!

Tom: You have collected quotes and sayings over the years to symbolize your life. Are there any you want to share?

Isaac:

God gives his toughest battles to his strongest soldiers.
– Habeeb Akande

Everything is going fine then one thing goes wrong.
Yet another and another until the harder
you fight the deeper you sink.
You can't move and you can't breathe
because you are in over your head.
You are stuck in quicksand.
(Taken from the 2000 Hollywood film "The Replacements"
by Bel Air Entertainment)

Let me show you another famous picture. It reads...

Hope for the best
Expect the worst
And take what comes.

I consider my present sufferings are not worth comparing to the glory that will be revealed in us. Romans 8:18

Tom: Any final thoughts?

Isaac: *After treatment at St. Jude, it took me awhile to figure some things in my new way of life. I know now my life is short, I gotta live life to the fullest, and don't take life too seriously because I will die someday. It's almost like I'm more alive now than I was before I had cancer.*

Tom: What do you mean as being more alive?

Isaac: *I'm more secure as a person now. I know who I am now, and it's changed my life. I don't live my life by what everyone thinks of me. Rather, I live my life by a quote from Dr. Seuss which reads...*

"Why fit in when you were born to stand out." – Dr. Seuss

Epilogue
Grey is the Color of Hope

The history of the cancer ribbon traces its beginnings to the Iran Hostage Crisis of the late 1970's. At the time, Penny Laingen whose husband was held captive in Iran, began tying yellow ribbons around her trees as a symbol of wanting to see her husband safely come home. Using the song, *"Tie a Yellow Ribbon Around the Old Oak Tree"* as an inspiration to show her solidarity with the nation's desire to see the release of the hostages, her actions soon became a nationwide movement. Today, a yellow ribbon is often tied around trees to show unity with US soldiers serving overseas.

Roughly ten years later, another group used bright red ribbons to represent awareness and support for the victims of AIDS. The trend caught on very quickly, with the New York Times declaring 1992 as the *"The Year of the Ribbon."* Further, it was also in 1992 the Susan G. Komen Breast Cancer Foundation started handing out pink hats to breast cancer survivors in their annual Race for the Cure event. Notwithstanding, it was at the same race everyone who participated was given a pink ribbon as a way to show support for their fellow racers who were cancer survivors. As the years went by more businesses and events began to use ribbons to raise an awareness of their cause.

In our present era, there are twenty-eight commonly recognized ribbons of cancer. The most popular ribbon is pink which is recognized by many to symbolize breast cancer. Further, the month of October is known as *Breast Cancer Awareness Month.* Another popular ribbon is orange which resembles a leukemia patient. Assigned to each form of cancer is/are a color(s) to signify the type of disease, and a month to raise awareness. However, some ribbons are made up of more than one color such as the ribbon for bladder cancer, which is blue, marigold and purple.

As for Isaac, grey is the color of his brain cancer ribbon. In addition, the month of May is known as brain cancer awareness month. Although rare, I sometimes see a grey ribbon at cancer events I attend. Often I see a purple *(plum)* colored ribbon which symbolizes a caregiver of a cancer survivor. For those who have fought the battle of cancer, the color assigned to their ribbon has become a symbol of courage.

St. Jude annually holds large fundraising events across the country in the month of September which is known as *Childhood Cancer Awareness Month*. It's also symbolized by a yellow ribbon. As for me, when Isaac and I participated in the St. Jude Walk to End Cancer event last fall, his grey ribbon symbolized more than the type of cancer he had. Rather, grey was the color of hope. A desire one day no one will need to wear a grey ribbon again.

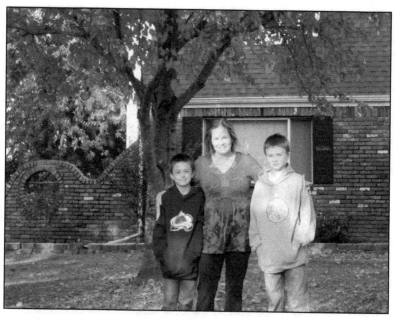

Prior to cancer treatments in November of 2010,
Dacia with the boys in our front yard.
From left to right: Caleb, Dacia and Isaac.

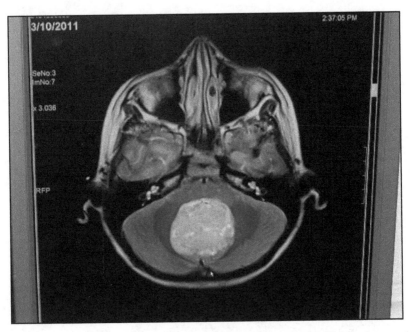

MRI scan dated March 10, 2011 showing the softball size
tumor lodged in Isaac's brain.
The nose is pictured at the top and ears to the side.

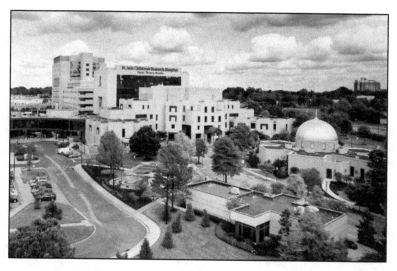

The sprawling campus of St. Jude Children's Research
Hospital in Memphis, Tennessee.
The Danny Thomas ALSAC Pavilion is marked by the gold
dome to the right in the photo.

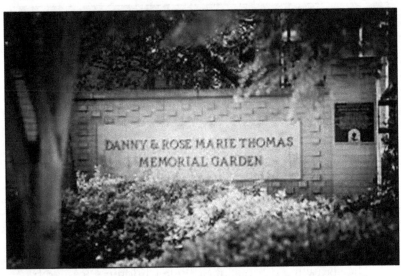

Three times during treatment I would visit the graveside
of Danny Thomas, *(Founder of St. Jude)*
as I contemplated life without my son Isaac.

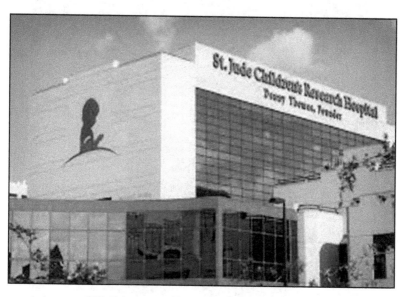

Visible to every visitor of St. Jude is
the image of a praying child.

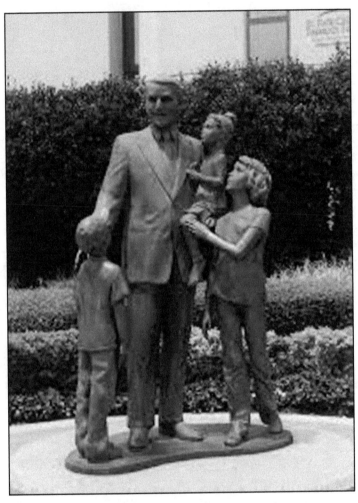

My favorite statue on the grounds of St. Jude is one of Danny Thomas surrounded by children. His life and dedication to finding a cure for cancer is an inspiration to me.

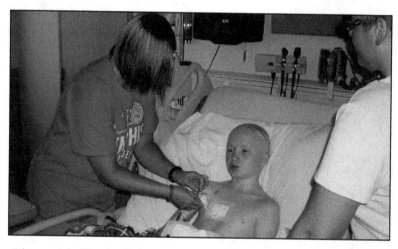
Pictured is Dacia disinfecting the double Hickman lines used to deliver chemotherapy drugs.

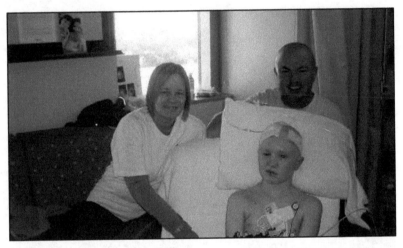

Pictured is Isaac after a ten-hour brain surgery in Memphis, Tennessee on April 6, 2011. It would be this surgery performed by St. Jude neurosurgeon Dr. Paul Klimo which would change the entire trajectory of treatment at St. Jude.

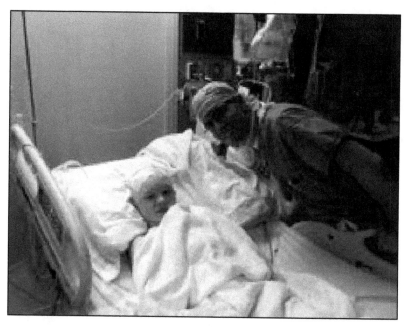

St. Jude neurosurgeon Dr. Paul Klimo pictured with Isaac
following surgery in April 2011.

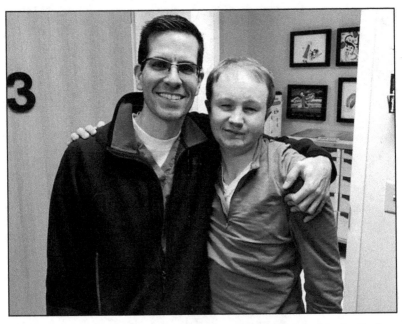

Isaac, at age 21 sharing a moment of gratitude with St. Jude neurosurgeon Dr. Paul Klimo.

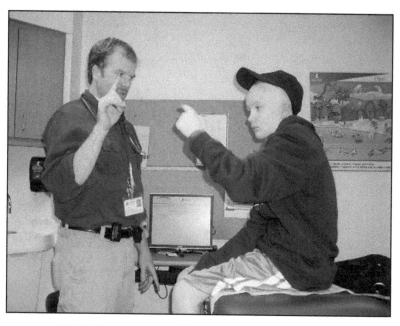

St. Jude neuro-oncologist Dr. Giles Robinson
administers a neuro exam to Isaac.

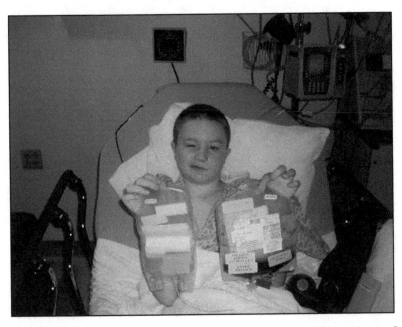

The start of cancer treatment at St. Jude. Isaac holding a bag of platelets and red blood cells prior to a transfusion.

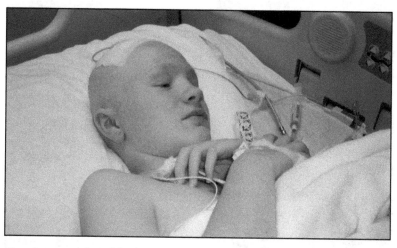

Resting comfortably is Isaac prior to the start of the first round
of chemotherapy in July 2011.

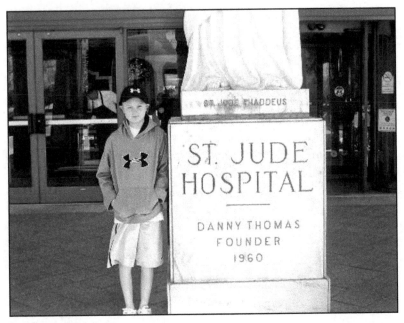

Isaac Walsh shortly after arrival at St. Jude in March 2011.

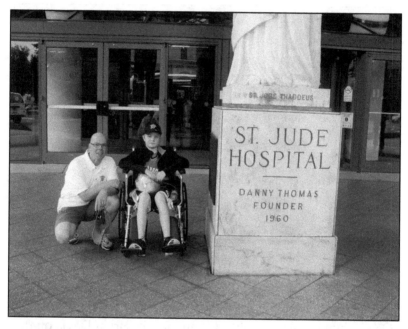

Oklahoma City play by play TV announcer Brian Davis with Isaac in May 2011.

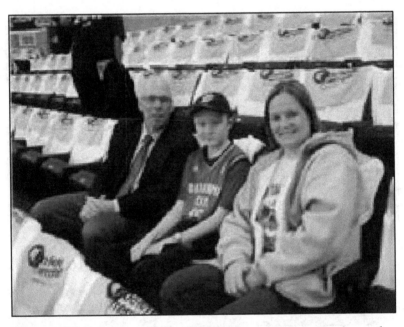

OKC Thunder play by play TV announcer Brian Davis on the night he walked up the arena at the FedEx Forum in downtown Memphis to meet Isaac.

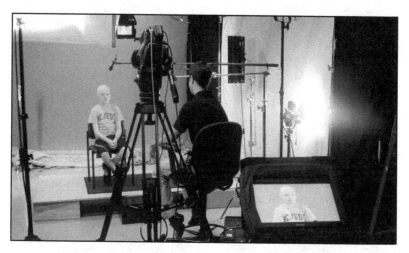

Isaac was interviewed for a fundraising story at St. Jude.

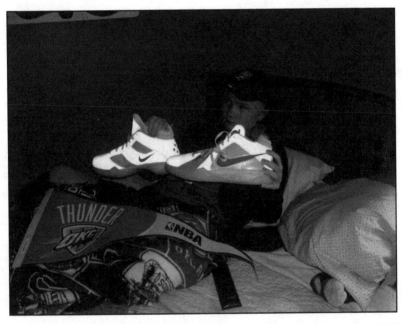

Compliments of Nicole Doyle were a pair of autographed OKC
Thunder forward Kevin Durant game shoes.

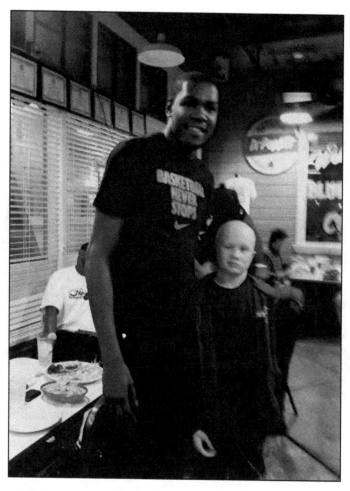

NBA superstar Kevin Durant pictured with Isaac at the Blues City Café on Memphis' Beale Street in November 2011.

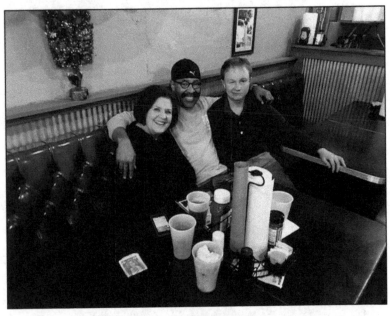

Blue City Café waiter Lonnie Yates and Memphis guardian
angel Juana McCoy pictured in March 2018.

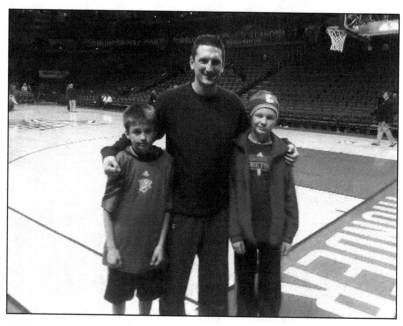

Oklahoma City Thunder assistant coach Nate Tibbetts pictured
with Caleb and Isaac Walsh.

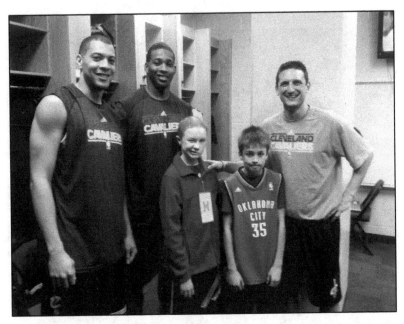

Former Oklahoma City Thunder and current Cleveland assistant coach Nate Tibbetts pictured here with Isaac and Caleb in the locker room of the visiting Cleveland Cavaliers at Chesapeake Arena in Oklahoma City during January 2013.

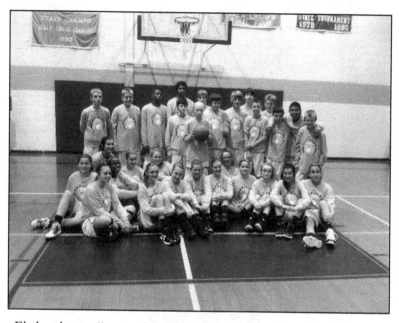

Fitting into a "normal," world as a recovering cancer patient would be the hardest thing I ever did according to Isaac Walsh. Pictured with Isaac are his former teammates in January 2012 only one month after being released from St. Jude.

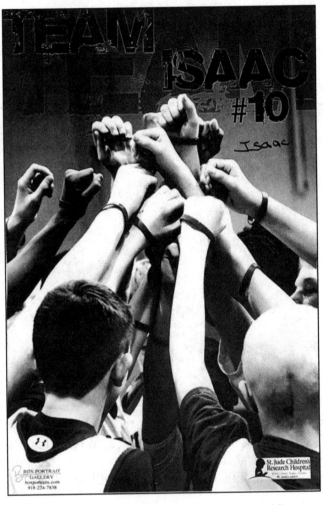

Photo creds: Pamela Jean ~ A New Life

Isaac is pictured here with his teammates during a basketball game in January 2012. This would be the final time Isaac wore a basketball jersey.

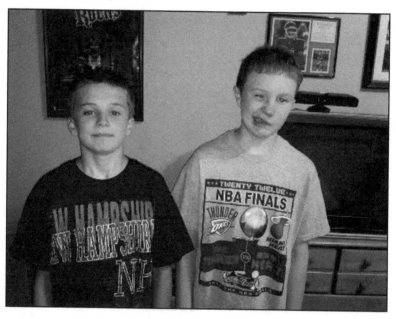

Isaac showing his trademark smile with his younger brother
Caleb after returning home in July 2012.

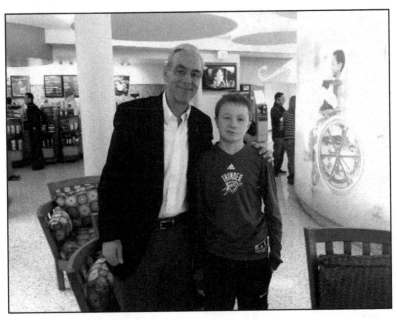

Wearing his Thunder gear, Isaac is pictured with St. Jude
ALSAC CEO Rick Shadyac in January 2015.

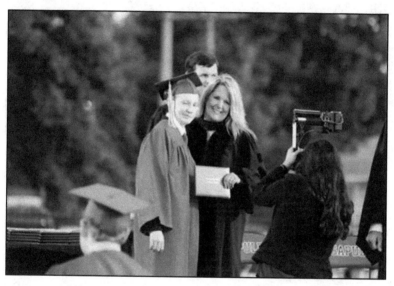

In this photo, Sapulpa Public Schools Board of Education President Melinda Ryan presents Isaac with his high school diploma in May 2016.

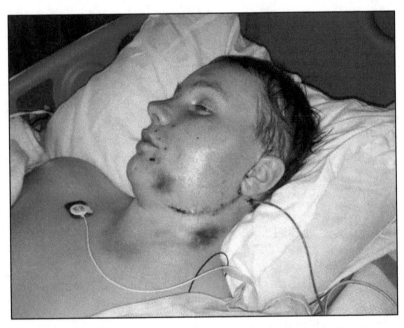

Isaac rests comfortably after a failed attempt at facial reanimation surgery in June 2018.

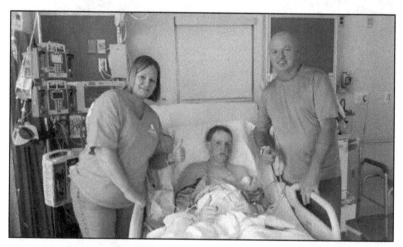

Isaac gives a "thumbs up" sign after learning his second attempt at restoring a smile nearly cost him his life in June 2018. This would be last of Isaac's twenty-one surgeries.

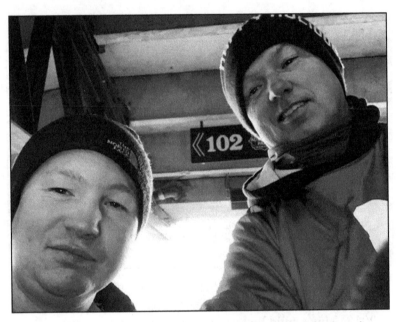

Father and son volunteering at the St. Jude Marathon in
December 2019.

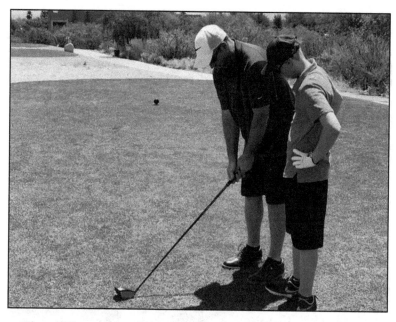

The ability to play basketball being gone, Isaac takes golf lessons from his Uncle Tim. Golf is one of the few sports which Isaac can play rather well.

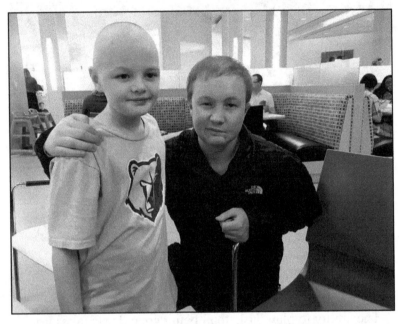

Once an employee at St. Jude ALSAC in the IT department, Isaac frequently met with young children undergoing cancer treatment.

Appendix

Compassion Came by the Hands of Devoted Family, Friends and Strangers

Reverend Mark Brown
Chaplain
St. Jude Children's Research Hospital

It was a busy day during our myriad of appointments upon our arrival at St. Jude in early April 2011. As we waited in an exam room for Isaac's oncologist, a very polite and cordial St. Jude Chaplain stopped by to introduce himself. He did not come across as someone wanting to intrude into a very personal aspect of our lives, rather, he demonstrated a tenderness towards our situation, and showed empathy towards our overwhelmed emotions. His words were encouraging, as his role was to both counsel and console families at a moment of hardship - which at times turned into loss. As our stay in Memphis grew into months, we formed a special friendship with St. Jude Chaplain Mark Brown.

Reverend Brown received his ordination from the Cumberland Presbyterian Church which is headquartered in Tennessee. Pastor Mark, as we came to call him, was a lifelong Memphian. He and his wife Elinor had one daughter Sydney, who recently gave birth to their first grandchild. It was through a mutual friend Sydney met her husband Brian, who works as a PHD microbiologist in a research tower at St. Jude. Prior to coming to St. Jude, Pastor Brown worked as a chaplain in an adult hospital located in Memphis. When asked what drew him to the children's cancer hospital only a few miles from his current place of employment, Reverend Brown explained he worked at St. Jude part-time for two years prior to permanently finding a home there. Pastor Mark remarked, "It was the love and compassion of the St. Jude staff that stood out the most to me during early years. When offered a fulltime job seventeen years ago, I gladly accepted." It would be the same kindness and empathy emulated by the work of Reverend Brown which led me to seek his advice after receiving news Isaac's life was about to come to an end.

We received a discouraging report about Isaac's condition following a major brain surgery at LeBonheur Children's Hospital. A staph infection had settled into his blood stream and a lifesaving follow-up surgery had been placed on hold. Dr. Klimo had been very direct when on a Wednesday morning he said, "If the staph infection does not start to clear by Thursday afternoon, call your friends and family. If they want to see Isaac alive before he passes, they must come before the weekend."

In my anguish and sorrow, I reached out to speak with Pastor Mark. Waiting for him in his office, my thoughts were erratic and confused. Isaac survived death once before in Tulsa and the thought of losing him now was more than I could stand. Gently closing the door, Reverend Brown listened with sympathy as I explained the devastating diagnosis we received from the doctors at LeBonheur Children's Hospital. Pastor Mark answered my cry for help with a spiritual insight which nine years later still inspires me. His response is noted below.

"God does a different miracle in the life of every child at St. Jude. There are some whom he calls home to be with him. These children are spared the radiation, chemotherapy and surgery as there is no cancer in heaven. For others, God uses his omnipotent power to send healing to their ailing bodies. Lastly, there are those for whom God uses the advancements made in

medicine today at St. Jude to send the cancer into remission. It's for this group, God also gives the parents the courage to help a child live a new life with the handicaps and disabilities the cancer treatment left behind."

Eight years later, I would recite the same compassionate words to a grieving mother whom I met at an NBA Washington Wizards basketball game at Capitol One Arena on a cold January night in 2019. Isaac and I had gone to the contest to see the Wizards take on the New York Knicks. My St. Jude apparel afforded me an opportunity to discuss Isaac's cancer treatments with a stranger seated beside us; a United States Air Force Major who worked at the Pentagon. During halftime, a young mother seated nearby timidly said she could not help but eavesdrop on our conversation. She and her husband lost their daughter to medulloblastoma brain cancer only one year prior. Diagnosed at age thirteen, their daughter initially survived only to succumb to a secondary tumor eight years later during college. She explained the heartache and grief which followed in the months since their daughter's passing. Reflecting back to Pastor Mark's conversation, I recited the same uplifting words he had given me years ago. When it was time for us to move back to our assigned arena seats, we stood up and gave each other a hug in a show of unity in our common bond. Fighting back tears, I realized I was not alone in my journey to find healing from the ravages of this dreadful disease.

It would be nine years after having met Pastor Mark that I found the courage to share with him the healing power of his words. Reverend Mark Brown has played a major role in the miracles happening at St. Jude. His work gave me hope when I was brokenhearted and healed my bruised emotions. I salute you Pastor Mark on being a true man of faith.

Dr. Mary Webb
Superintendent (Ret.)
Sapulpa Public Schools

Leaving Oklahoma for what would be the start of her forty-year career in education, a young college graduate from Oklahoma State University decided to move with a fellow sorority sister to start a new life in Central City, Colorado. The young girls did not have jobs prior to relocating to the Rocky Mountains. Rather, the allure of cool crisp air and a chance to set their own course in life led them to this new adventure. The girls were elated when one week prior to the start of school they got hired as teachers in Jefferson County Public Schools. One of the two would only last five years before relocating back to her hometown, Sapulpa, Oklahoma. Mary Webb would decide to come home.

Mary was immediately hired as a seventh grade English teacher at the town's only middle school. Teaching for only seven years, Mary decided to work on her master's degree and later a PHD at the University of Tulsa. As for me, I became acquainted with Dr. Mary Webb when she was hired as the Sapulpa Public Schools Director of Secondary Curriculum in 1992. Dr. Webb reached the pinnacle of her career when in 2008 she was hired to be the Superintendent of Sapulpa Public Schools. This would be a tumultuous time as the financial crisis which besieged our country saw the loss of funding for Oklahoma public schools. Guiding Sapulpa through this chaotic time was a challenge unlike Mary had ever faced in life. Letting her commitment to teachers be her guide, Mary coveted the opinions of others and marshalled all competing sides to gain a consensus to fend off the loss of jobs. Looming on the horizon only two years later, a principal's son was diagnosed with medulloblastoma brain cancer. The disease would ripple through the small community of Sapulpa bringing an abysmal sense of despair to all who knew Sapulpa Middle School student Isaac Walsh.

I found myself at the crossroads of trying to resolve how to best provide for my family and exist in a time of profound crisis. Isaac's cancer diagnosis left me feeling powerless to control the outcome this illness would bring. The reality of a near year-long treatment protocol yielded fears of how our family could financially survive. How could we juggle our jobs as educators and be with our son in Memphis, nearly four hundred miles from home? Should we stay in Tulsa knowing the possibility of severe brain damage the cancer treatments would leave in its wake?

On the night of March 9th in the lobby of St. Francis Children's Hospital, something happened which became the first miracle in our long journey with cancer. A large gathering of at least one hundred people assembled to show their support and compassion on the day of Isaac's tumor resection surgery. Overwhelmed with the heartache of Isaac's diagnosis, I went to the lobby to greet those who had patiently waited well into the evening hours. Coming to greet me as I walked into the reception area was my superintendent, Dr. Mary Webb. I will never forget her empathetic words, "Tom, you will have whatever you need from me. Take care of your family. You will have a job to come back to once Isaac comes home."

Nine years later when I met with Dr. Webb, the same compassionate condolences were there as she said, "In a district this size, we were family. We look out for each other and most importantly – family comes first." Dr. Webb remained true to her promise. Nine years ago the Sapulpa Board of Education voted to allow Dacia to access a donation of sick leave from fellow employees. Unlike anything seen in the Sapulpa school district, Dacia received 180 days or what would be the equivalent to an entire year of paid leave as a result of her colleagues generous giving. Further, Dr. Webb allowed me to utilize my sick leave and to spend the entire ten months with Isaac at St. Jude. Just as Dr. Webb had pledged, one year later I returned to my job as principal at Jefferson Heights Elementary School. Dacia would return to her work as a Title I Reading Teacher at Holmes Park Elementary, working in the morning hours while Isaac attended school.

I commend Dr. Mary Webb for an unyielding commitment to the value of family. It was through her benevolent leadership my family was saved from financial ruin. Further, Isaac was able to have both parents by his side throughout the entire course of treatment at St. Jude. Dr. Webb you are a part of the reason our family survived this dreadful disease. We are forever grateful.

Jennifer Poyner
Senior Advisor – Special Projects and Integration
ALSAC/St. Jude Children's Research Hospital

In 2004, ALSAC, the fundraising and awareness organization for St. Jude Children's Research Hospital hired a recent journalism major from the University of Memphis. Previously, she had worked as the volunteer coordinator at a local non-profit. This young professional wanted to find a career which would blend her writing talents with service to children. Scanning the job postings in the local newspaper, she decided to apply for a job with the patient outreach team at ALSAC. Jennifer Poyner was one of three hundred applicants considered, and the only one hired that day. Seven years later, Jennifer would cross my path when she held the position of patient outreach director.

I formed a friendship with Jennifer which lasted long after we returned home to Oklahoma. She became more than just a professional ALSAC worker from the fundraising department but a trusted friend. In my discussion with Jennifer, as I prepared the writing of this book, I asked what's the biggest challenge she faces while working at St. Jude? Her response echoed what I felt nine years ago when she said, "This is the most intense emotional crisis in a family's life. You must be driven to serve others and have your heart in the right place."

It did not take the staff at St. Jude long to realize Isaac was an NBA basketball fan. Every day he would wear his Oklahoma City Thunder apparel and fan gear through the halls of the hospital. Realizing the pathway to Isaac's heart was through sports, Jennifer began to arrange meetings from sports celebrities visiting the hospital. In a small and sincere way, this helped Isaac reclaim his life as the athlete the cancer had stripped away. I remember a visit with training staff of the NBA's Philadelphia 76er's arranged by Jennifer. The team was in town for a basketball game with the Memphis Grizzlies at the FedEx Forum. The young group of medical doctors, trainers and therapists wanted to reach out and meet a patient's family. I was captivated by their kindness and the questions each one asked. Our conversation was more than just why are you here and what type of cancer do you have? Rather, the team dietician asked what his favorite food was at St. Jude – burgers! More so, they asked about school and his family. Isaac explained he had a younger brother who could not be with him while he was undergoing treatment at St. Jude. As it always happened with Isaac, the conversation quickly turned to the players, the game stats and the outlook of the playoffs. The lead trainer tugged me aside and wanted to know if they could send both boys some 76'ers souvenirs. I offered their shirt sizes but explained the gifts would have to go through proper channels of the ALSAC division of the hospital. Roughly two weeks later came two official 76'er jerseys fitted to a smaller size, sweat bands, mini basketballs, team socks and an autographed team picture for each child.

Working in the fundraising and awareness organization for the hospital, Jennifer embodies the same compassionate care we felt from the medical staff at St. Jude. She is part of the reason kids like Isaac are afforded the same opportunities in life as those who never face the scourge of cancer at a young age. Today, Jennifer works in the Marketing division of ALSAC. In her wheelhouse are the St. Jude Memphis Marathon, St. Jude Walk/Run to End Childhood Cancer and the World Golf Championships-FedEx St. Jude Invitational to name just a few of the many fundraising events held each year. In this roll, Jennifer is the unsung hero many patient families will never meet.

For the past nine years a picture of Isaac returning to the basketball court hung in my office at school. In the picture,

Isaac is joined by his teammates all wearing TEAM Isaac bracelets with their hands lifted high during a timeout. The citation reads...

> *"You never know how strong you are until being strong is the only choice you have."* – *Anonymous*

Please know Jennifer, you are part of the reason Isaac agreed to play a celebratory role in a basketball game only one month after being released from treatment at St. Jude. He came with the battle marks of cancer – a six-inch visible scar on his bald head and an uncoordinated ability to run. As his jump shot went through the hoop, a crooked smile appeared on his face as he walked back to the bench. The crowd cheered and gave him a five-minute standing ovation. As for me, I thought about you. Your ability to connect Isaac with those whom he idolized in sports gave him the strength he never knew he had.

Juana McCoy
Retired Small Business Owner and Guardian Angel
Memphis, Tennessee

In the checkout line at Walgreens in Midtown Memphis, Isaac's uncovered head revealed the surgery scars to all who were around us. As I handed the credit card to the clerk, she asked for our zip code as it was a customary security procedure at the time. Standing closely behind us was a lifelong retired Memphian who knew a bald child with surgery scars must be a patient at St. Jude. Asking if we had family in town and soon realizing we were strangers to the city of Memphis; she became persistent in wanting to get our contact information. Reluctantly, I remember writing down our phone numbers on a piece of paper for this stranger. At the time, I never really thought much of it. However, I had no idea of how persistent this person would be to help. Recalling the encounter nine years later, she would say "It hit me unexpectedly like a bucket of water to the face. They cannot go through this alone. I simply cannot let it happen." A week later she and Dacia had lunch together. Soon thereafter, I met her for lunch at Central BBQ and later welcomed her for the first time to the grounds of St. Jude. She was someone who would share in joys and grieve when the outlook became grim – Juana McCoy had become our guardian angel.

Juana was born and raised in Memphis, TN. Ms. McCoy graduated from Stephens College in Columbia, Missouri with a degree in comparative literature back in the 1960's. It was during this time Juana lost her husband in a small plane crash over the high plains of western Texas. In an instant, Juana's life was tragically changed as she became a single parent to her only son Robert. Upon returning to Memphis, she opened two retail stores which sold high end cosmetics. Juana would run the business until the financial crisis of 2007. To our family,

Juana McCoy was more than a stranger whom we met at Walgreens – she soon became family.

Juana recalled a night at St. Jude when she was staying with Isaac. Dacia and I had gone out for dinner to celebrate our anniversary. A doctor came by the room and asked Isaac who this older lady was with him. Isaac did not flinch but answered directly by saying, "She is my grandma." Years later Juana, Isaac and I were having dinner on her front porch and she would add, "I wanted to cry. I worked on this title a long time. This meant the world to me."

As with any loving paternal bond, Juana saw Isaac through his worst days. She was there with him during the chemotherapy rounds marked by fevers of 106 and changed his sheets when he was nauseous. Grandma Juana earned her place in our family as a caregiver, friend and most importantly as someone who rescued us at our time of greatest need. We said goodbye to Juana McCoy on December 21, 2011 after being released from St. Jude. However, in the years which followed we would visit her on every trip to St. Jude for checkup visits in the clinical trial. Juana would be called upon again when her grandson accepted a job at St. Jude Children's Research Hospital in the IT department on June 1, 2018.

Juana arranged a garage apartment for Isaac to rent from a retired elementary school principal in an upscale neighborhood ten minutes from the hospital. Juana recalled the times Isaac would come over to her house on Sundays to do his laundry. Food would be ready, and during the fall football would be on TV. Many a weekend Isaac would go to Juana's house to watch football and take a nap. Never once did he do his own laundry – Grandma Juana took care of it all.

Today, I look back on the day we met Juana in Walgreens and smile. Juana embodies a faithful servant who took it upon herself to become our guardian angel. I can only think the founder of St. Jude had her in mind when he said…

"All of us are born for a reason, but all of us don't discover why. Success in life has nothing to do with what you gain in life or accomplish for yourself. It's what you do for others." – Danny Thomas (Founder of St. Jude Children's Research Hospital)

As for me, I will forever be grateful to this wonderful woman who came into our family. When I think of Memphis – I will always remember Juana McCoy's act of compassion which transformed our lives four hundred miles from home.

James Womack
Former Sapulpa High School Varsity Head Coach
Boys Basketball Team

The sound of a dribbled basketball echoed throughout the gym. Each Saturday a large group of parents cheered as they watched their children compete in a recreational church basketball league. Some boys arched shots which had no chance of even coming close to hitting the rim. Yet, their parents would cheer as if it were the game winning shot made at the buzzer in a championship game. Some unskilled players were not able to dribble the ball and instead ran as if it were a prized toy they were trying to keep from their younger siblings. Each time the Walsh boy got the ball everyone's head would turn. His long three-point shots would make it almost every time, and no one was any match for his defensive skills. Isaac Walsh was the star of his little league team. His basketball prowess soon caught the eye of Sapulpa High School varsity boys' basketball head coach James Womack.

It was summer and time for the traditional start of athletic camps. Isaac and his younger brother Caleb were attending a basketball camp put on by the Sapulpa High School boys' varsity head coach James Womack. Isaac was in fifth grade and still five years from his high school career. However, Isaac's ability to play sports was something which immediately caught Coach Womack's attention. "Isaac had a cool and calm collectiveness about him. His skill set was advanced for someone his age. One can go down the basketball fundamental checklist and Isaac had it all." Coach Womack saw more than just a talented player in this young athlete when he said, "Isaac could play under pressure. He had the mental toughness to be a leader among his teammates." Coach Womack would talk with his assistants about the grooming and coaching this future star athlete would need to be a leader in their program. However,

149

during Isaac's seventh grade year, tragedy struck and his future as a high school basketball star was cast in doubt.

Coach Womack recalled the day he found out one of his elementary age stars had been admitted to the hospital with a brain tumor. At first, he recalled his quick denial in thinking this isn't serious. Isaac was only a kid and in a short amount of time he would be back in school. However, more testing would reveal Isaac had a softball size malignant brain tumor which had a dismal survivor record. Coach Womack recalled his confused emotions by saying, "This was a life ending illness which could happen to anyone." Painfully he would remember thinking, "How could this happen? This is not the same person I watched through the years playing basketball."

Coach Womack remembers the day Isaac arrived in high school. He was uncoordinated and had a large six-inch scar down the back of his head. His ability to shoot the ball was no longer on par with his peers nor was his ability to dribble down the court. However, Coach Womack noticed one thing about Isaac which had not changed - the mental toughness and ability to think under pressure was something the cancer did not strip away. Coach Womack later approached me with the idea of bringing Isaac on as a manager of the team. He also wanted to know what the doctors at St. Jude had recommended in terms of his approved fitness activities, and what he could participate in, in terms of team drills. Dacia and I were excited about this new opportunity and said Isaac was free to do any workouts the team did. He was old enough to be the best judge of his pain.

Coach Womack soon approached Isaac about joining the team as a manager. Isaac gladly accepted the offer, but it came with one condition. Coach Womack later recalled what he told Isaac, "This is not a charity case. You are not going to come in and stand around. You will work out every day with your teammates." Coach Womack would reminisce about Isaac when he said, "He did not want to be put on display, he just wanted to be a normal guy. I wanted to give him back his basketball identity." Isaac would do the workouts with his fellow players. Coach Womack recalled one drill which involved jumping from the floor to a sturdy bench. Isaac had worked unsuccessfully on the skill for months but one day the entire team gathered around and cheered him on. Unskilled and with little coordination in his legs – Isaac made it. Coach Womack put it best when he said, "He served as an incredible inspiration of what you want a champion to be."

Coach Womack gave Isaac one of the greatest gifts he received throughout his entire ordeal with cancer, a chance to be treated as a normal kid in a world which did not understand what he had been through. More so, Coach Womack taught others to value him, not for his athletic accomplishments, but rather for an undeterred passion which had faced death in the eye and did not lose its will to live. As for me, Coach Womack represents more than just someone who wanted to help Isaac adjust after coming home. He demonstrated, through treating those less fortunate with the same pride and respect we give our star athletes; we can create a culture where disabilities and handicaps are prized for the strength it takes to overcome them. Although Isaac never played in a high school game, I'm glad he got a chance to be a player under the leadership of this legendary coach. In much humility and respect, Coach Womack would only say, "Isaac did more for me than I did for him." As coaches frequently do, he ended our conversation with a Shakespearian quote which not only spoke so well of Isaac but inspires me to be a better person.

Great Men, Hard Times, Must Endure – Isaac Walsh

Nate Tibbetts
Associate Head Coach of the NBA Portland Trailblazers
Portland, Oregon

Growing up in a small town of five hundred people on the northern high plains of South Dakota, a young boy dreamed of becoming an NBA basketball coach. Not a usual route for coaches at the highest professional level, he grew up a "gym rat," as his family lived next door to the high school gymnasium. In a state known for its winter sport of hockey, this young man became a star in an indoor arena, far from the cold northern winds. He would start all four years of high school as a point guard, and in his senior year earn all-state honors. Recruited by a local university to play collegiate basketball near his hometown, Nate Tibbetts began his long journey to coach in the NBA.

Nate aspired to be like his dad, Fred Tibbetts who was a South Dakota Hall of Fame legendary high school girls' basketball coach. Coach Tibbetts coaching record was 551 – 101 over twenty-nine seasons. His teams would reach state finals fifteen times and win eleven titles. Notwithstanding, seven of teams won the state championship without losing a game all season long. Coach Tibbitts would form a special bond with his son who shared his love of basketball. Upon graduation from the University of Sioux Falls, Nate took a head coaching job with the NBA developmental league affiliate in his hometown – the Sioux Falls Skyforce. His dad would attend every game and call when the team was away. Like many coaches at the professional level, the coaching carousel would stop in Tulsa, Oklahoma. Nate took over head coaching duties for a team affiliated with the Oklahoma City Thunder, known as the Tulsa 66er's. Tragedy would overtake Tibbetts family when Fred Tibbetts was diagnosed with colon cancer. Fred Tibbetts would never get to see his son coach in the NBA, as he succumbed to the disease on February 19, 2008. He was only fifty-eight years old when he died.

I met Nate Tibbetts when we took Isaac to see the visiting Oklahoma City Thunder take on the Memphis Grizzlies in the NBA playoffs on May 10, 2011. Squeamishly, I walked into the arena abuzz with the rancor of the playoffs with a child wearing an OKC Thunder jersey. Before the game I walked down to the floor in an unsuccessful effort to get a player's attention. However, I recognized the OKC Thunder TV announcer who eagerly came up into the arena to meet Isaac. He told Isaac he wanted him to meet someone else, a few minutes later we met Nate Tibbetts. Both men were very gracious and demonstrated compassion towards Isaac. We exchanged phone numbers with a promise to reconnect soon. Recalling the event nine years later, Coach Tibbetts would say, "Seeing you and your wife in the arena and knowing the challenges you were about to face, hit me probably the hardest." Nate's kindness did not end at the conclusion of the game. When Nate was named head coach of Team USA during the 2011 Pan-American Games in Guadalajara, Mexico, the boys received *(in the mail)* Team USA backpacks complete with hats, sweatbands, arm sleeves and towels. One year later, Nate took an assistant coaching job with the NBA Cleveland Cavaliers, yet his outreach to the boys continued. We had gone to the arena in Oklahoma City to see Nate Tibbett's team take on our OKC Thunder. Before the game, Nate walked into the stands and got both boys. Leading them passed security, they greeted the Cleveland players on the court and walked past a long line of adoring fans lining the tunnel to the team locker room. Roughly twenty minutes later both boys walked out of the tunnel with team towels, wristbands, autographs and memories which would last a lifetime.

Nine years later, I would discuss this game with my youngest son Caleb who is now twenty years old. Finding it difficult to speak and holding back his emotions Caleb said, "It's every child's dream to go out onto the court and meet the players. Never does anyone get to go into the locker room. It gave me hope that our life might be normal again." As for Isaac, he cherishes the souvenirs, and for nine years has followed Nate's career. He could recite the list of teams who brought Coach Tibbetts in for an interview for their head coaching position. Isaac would joke, "I was always a Trailblazer fan because Nate was there. However, when they beat the Thunder in the playoffs several years ago. I quit following them."

Reflecting upon his life as a father now, Nate said, "I'm glad those things were a positive in your life at such a difficult time. I knew you had some dark days ahead of you. It's difficult to read Isaac almost died three times. Now having kids of my own it's hard to fathom what it must have been like." Nate told me nine years ago after losing his father to cancer a part of him was changed forever. The death of a parent at a young age is one of the most tragic things in life a child has to face. Nate had developed a close relationship with his dad - much like two best friends. The loss would crush his spirit and linger for years to come. As for me, the day I met Nate Tibbetts a part of my life changed as well. Realizing by extending an empathetic hand to others, I too could heal. Soon thereafter, I began sharing our story by speaking at various fundraising events at St. Jude. I noticed my life was being transformed as I reached out to others in my brokenness. Nate's compassion towards both my children was an example of what represents the best in our sport's celebrities. More so, Nate's willingness to bless others in his greatest time of need is an example I strive to follow to this day.

The NBA Cares
Memphis, TN

Both our boys growing up were always sports fans. The love of the game was more than just watching the contests on TV. Rather, Isaac and Caleb enjoyed going to collegiate football and basketball games. For many years, there were no major professional sports teams based in Oklahoma. However, when the NBA's Seattle Supersonics were purchased by Oklahoma businessman Clay Bennett, the landscape of pro sports in Oklahoma changed. Mr. Bennett relocated the Seattle franchise to Oklahoma City with a new nickname, the Oklahoma City Thunder. Isaac instantly became their biggest fan. He would follow the team trades, statistics and games on a daily basis. He was known throughout the hospital as the OKC Thunder boy who daily wore the team jersey and proudly supported his team.

St. Jude has a strong partnership with sports celebrities and professional basketball teams in the NBA. During our stay at St. Jude, Isaac met Pau Gasol who at the time played for the Los Angeles Lakers. Pau's visit was part of an outreach to the Hispanic community and was being filmed for public service announcements on CNN en Espanol and Telemundo. Pau was very kind and gracious towards Isaac. He signed some autographs and demonstrated genuine compassion in learning about the side effects of cancer treatment on young children. As a special present for Isaac, St. Jude ALSAC CEO Rick Shadyac worked out an arrangement for Isaac and family to see the Memphis Grizzlies host the Los Angeles Lakers at the FedEx Forum. The owner of the Grizzlies had heard about Pao's visit with Isaac and wanted to show compassion as well, he donated his own seats for us to view the game.

We found within the Memphis community a strong appreciation for the work of St. Jude. During the course of our time in Memphis, we frequently visited Memphis' Beale Street as we really enjoyed eating at the Blues City Café. We quickly became friends with a waiter named Lonnie Yates who told us visiting NBA teams would often frequent the restaurant during their time in Memphis. Lonnie became a trusted friend who followed Isaac's diagnosis with cancer from our first month in Memphis until present day. Isaac presented Lonnie with a picture of himself taken at St. Jude which is now prominently displayed among all the professional NBA sports stars at the restaurant. Lonnie knew of Isaac's love for the Oklahoma City Thunder. He monitored the NBA games and player stats as religiously as Isaac did. Each time we would come to the restaurant they would talk about the outlook for the playoffs, which team would be next in Memphis, etc. When the NBA and its players union reached an impasse during the summer of our chemotherapy treatment, all off season workouts came to a screeching halt. In effect, the league shut down.

The NBA lockout would last from July 1, 2011 – December 8, 2011. The traditional start of the NBA season would come and go without any games being played in late October. Isaac got excited when some NBA players announced they would be playing in a charity basketball game hosted by Rudy Gay of the Memphis Grizzlies at the Desoto Civic Center *(Mississippi)* on Tuesday, November 8, 2011. Many of the NBA stars would be in attendance including the Cleveland Cavaliers forward Lebron James and OKC Thunder forward Kevin Durant.

Isaac was at a critical juncture during cancer treatment. He was doing his chemotherapy rounds, and his blood counts were being monitored on a daily basis. The blood marker which determined what Isaac was able to do outside the hospital was his immune system value. I will never forget the oncologist's words to Isaac the night before the game, "Isaac, I'm truly sorry but your blood counts are too low for you to be in a large crowd of people at a basketball game. My advice to your parents is you stay away due to the risk it poses for you." The doctor's words crushed Isaac's fragile spirit and left him with a feeling of dejection reminiscent of when he first learned he had cancer. As a parent, I felt hopeless knowing we could ignore the doctor's counsel to appease Isaac, but the end result could prove fatal for him. I suggested and the doctor concurred we go to the Blues City Café on Beale Street and see our waiter Lonnie. Resentful and dejected, Isaac agreed to go.

I dropped Isaac and Dacia off at the front door to the restaurant. The damp cold air reminded me of the holiday season, yet it provided no solace as I knew this would be a difficult night for Isaac. At the time, Isaac received all his nutritional needs *(food)* through a large bag of fluids which were infused through his double Hickman lines. He wore a backpack to carry the IV bags, and always kept a hat on his head to hide the surgery scars. Watching his mom and dad eat a steak dinner was no substitute for his dream of seeing OKC Thunder forward Kevin Durant playing in the charity game. Our waiter Lonnie had become a source of encouragement to Isaac. Hopefully, Lonnie's ability to communicate with Isaac by telling him stories of the NBA stars who visited the restaurant, would erase some of the bitter disappointment Isaac felt. We did not know it at the time, but an NBA basketball player had come to Blues City at the same time we were there. As was customary, the wait staff shielded him from autograph seekers and gave his party privacy in a secluded area of the restaurant.

Lonnie came to the table and asked if we were ready for dessert. He chided Isaac about not eating anything and joked maybe what he could offer next would be better than a double fudge brownie and ice cream. Isaac politely smiled and said,

"No thanks." Lonnie persisted and asked Isaac to follow him to an area of the restaurant we rarely visited. Standing to greet us was a large 6'11" forward with the Oklahoma City Thunder named Kevin Durant. Isaac was overjoyed and could hardly contain his emotions. Most of the wait staff at the restaurant had gathered to see a cancer-stricken child's dream fulfilled by meeting his sports idol. As Isaac shook Kevin Durant's large hand, I could only smile as I thought the doctor had prescribed this visit himself.

I had the opportunity to speak in great detail with the NBA star about the cancer treatments being done at St. Jude. I vividly remember his words when he saw Isaac's six-inch surgery on the back of his head where the tumor had been removed. Somewhat stunned Kevin Durant remarked, "It's not fair, he's only a kid." The OKC Thunder forward did not disappoint when he signed numerous souvenirs the staff had put together for Isaac. I looked over at Lonnie and saw a prized smile. He had joined the ranks of those who were part of the miracles which occurred in Isaac's young life. Kevin Durant was wearing a t-shirt with the words, "Basketball Never Stops." I could only grin as we left the restaurant thinking Lonnie had given us the true meaning of professional basketball – "The NBA Cares."

Meri Armour
President *(Ret.)*
Le Bonheur Children's Hospital
Memphis, Tennessee

In 1973 Meri Armour went to work as a nurse at Ohio State University Medical Center in the field of oncology. Her childhood dream was to be a nurse, but as often happens her career took another turn. She went back to school and ten years later earned a master's degree in nursing from the Francis Payne Bolton School of Nursing. In addition, Meri paired her medical talents with a degree in business administration from Weatherford School of Management associated with Case Western Reserve University. Moving with her husband Don to Cleveland in 1987, Meri went to work as a nurse at the Cleveland Clinic. It was during this time Meri began a transition from nursing to hospital administration. Meri would be instrumental in starting the pediatric oncology program at Cleveland Clinic. Soon thereafter on the heels of the children's cancer program was her work with the establishment of the Rainbow Baby & Children's Hospital Cancer Center and the Ronald McDonald House.

I first became acquainted with Meri Armour through the work of the nurses at Le Bonheur Children's Hospital in Memphis, Tennessee. St. Jude has a close partnership with Le Bonheur, as many doctors work at both hospitals. Le Bonheur is also a trauma care center with a wide array of specialties and highly trained nursing staff. It's for this reason, St. Jude completes many surgeries at their sister hospital located only a mile from their front door. My first interaction with the Le Bonheur nursing staff would parallel my impression of the employees of St. Jude – a high standard of excellence combined with compassion. More than one nurse would tell me they were a former employee at St. Jude. Perplexed, I would ask their reason for leaving and each time garner the same answer. St. Jude specialized in oncology and it was too hard to see families in a time of such sorrow and pain. Cancer came with a life and death consequence and for some the outcome of this kind of work was too harrowing and arduous to endure. However, there was something special about the nurses at Le Bonheur. Most had a cordial working relationship with the boss – President Meri Armour.

I first met Meri Armour after a complicated hospital stay, in what for Isaac was a smile reanimation elective surgery. Isaac underwent a twenty-five hour microsurgery to transplant a muscle from his inner thigh to the paralyzed side of his face. Due to blood clotting, the twelve-day exhaustive procedure failed. St. Jude would later determine after a comprehensive several month study of Isaac's DNA, the failure of the operation was due to his body rejecting the muscle graph. The team at Le Bonheur was heartbroken as Isaac's smile could not be restored. I was told nurses would often call on their days off to check on Isaac's condition. Further, I witnessed during this time an incredible spirit of teamwork and unity on the part of the entire team. I remember one night when the head plastic surgeon spent the entire night by Isaac's side, dressing his wounds and monitoring the blood flow in the transplanted muscle. Throughout the night, eighteen blood transfusions had to be given. Nurses willingly gave up their dinner breaks to assist the nurse assigned to our room. In my twenty-four years as school principal, I never witnessed such an act of unselfish compassion and love, by a team of professionals. It was at heart, medical care delivered at its best.

A good friend told me early in my career, "Organizations rise and fall based on leadership. The most successful leaders are able to attract the best talent and retain their finest employees." His words to me were even more pointed when he said, "You will share in their success, but you must embrace one hidden truth – failure will be a direct result of your leadership." As for me, this was best exemplified in the life of President Meri Armour.

Meri told me once going to *"church"* for her was visiting the hospital floors on Sunday morning. Reflecting back to her roots as a nurse, Meri would develop and foster an attitude of cooperation by telling nurses, "Your job is to take care the entire family. People in a children's hospital come as a package deal. The entire family will be affected by the work you do here today." Meri's compassion and nurturing words did not occur only on Sundays. While interviewing Meri for the writing of this book she remarked, "If it was a long day of meetings and budget sessions, I would recess the meeting and take sixty minutes to visit the families on the floor." This visual example of servant leadership would develop and train medical professionals when care went wrong. Meri's attitude towards failure was to learn from mistakes, and for leadership to determine what supports were needed to prevent the problem from occurring again.

During Meri's twelve-year tenure as President, the hospital would win accolades from US World & News Report's ranking of hospital specialties, and see the renovation of the entire facility. When Meri retired in 2019, the Le Bonheur Board of Directors established the *Legacy of Promise: Meri Armour Fund* to secure the hospital's $100 million endowment, which will secure the hospital's future.

I will always remember Meri's commitment to the children and families who came to her hospital seeking care. Her compassionate interactions with staff and willingness to stay true to her early beginnings as a nurse made a lasting impression on me. We all should strive to be a Meri Armour. I'm forever grateful for the short time our paths intersected and the friendship we now share. President Armour represented the best of healthcare practitioners, and blessed are those who worked under her leadership.

Joan Eisenstodt
President and Founder of Eisenstodt Associates LLC
Washington D.C.

In every person's life there comes a time when a stranger performs a random act of kindness which reaffirms in us the goodness of mankind. As a principal at an elementary school in an impoverished area of town, we had an Angel Tree set up in our hallway during the December holidays. Unselfishly and sometimes with very little money to spare, many of my teachers would "adopt," children in their own classrooms not wanting them to feel the rejection of waking up on this special day without any presents. Their students rejoiced and played with toys wrapped by the hand of an anonymous angel - often their very own teacher. The stranger who took our "angel," card from the tree, established when Isaac befell to cancer, was Joan Eisenstodt.

Joan grew up in Dayton, Ohio and hailed from a military family. Joan's mother drove a jeep on Wright-Patterson Air Force Base during World War II while her dad served overseas. This was the same base where Dr. Paul Klimo was stationed with the 88th Medical Air Wing during Operation Enduring Freedom in Afghanistan. Throughout the duration of WWII, Joan's family invited Jewish airmen from the base to their home during the month of Passover. Joan's commitment to her Jewish roots reaffirmed the example set by her parents – service to others is key to happiness.

Joan would not spend her working years in Dayton, Ohio. She told me she visited Washington DC once and fell in love with the city. She recalls, "I had a job interview in DC and got turned down. So, I moved anyway and volunteered at the very company who did not want me." Forty-two years later Joan owns a hospitality consulting company which works with local venues to bring in conferences and annual company meetings.

I've never met Joan in person and up until the writing of this book never spoke with her over the phone. Meeting with Joan through a Zoom interview on June 30, 2020 was reminiscent of a reunion with a distant family member whom you never knew. Nevertheless, our encounter was warm and friendly. The conversation flowed as if we had been friends our entire lives. Like a small child who gets to meet the "angel," who gave them a bicycle on Christmas Day, I finally met Joan.

Joan came to know our family through a distant connection with another St. Jude Oklahoma family. Like many St. Jude families, we established a Caring Bridge social media website soon after Isaac's diagnosis. I updated the site daily to keep our friends and family informed as to Isaac's condition and outlook. In the comments section of the website, we noticed kind words of warmth and well wishes from someone in Washington D.C. named Joan Eisenstodt. We got an email from her wanting to know our address in Memphis, as she read on our Caring Bridge site Isaac would be celebrating his birthday while going through chemotherapy. A week later an Amazon gift card arrived along with some Oklahoma City Thunder apparel. Joan's generosity did not end with Isaac. Mindful of the aching heart of a younger brother four hundred miles from his family, gifts arrived for Caleb too.

I remember the day I wrote on our Caring Bridge site about shaving Isaac's head due to the onset of radiation. Joan posted in the comments section her concerns and said there would be something coming our way – an OKC Thunder baseball hat arrived a few days later. During the winter months, Joan mailed stocking caps and beanies. Her heartfelt comments on our Caring Bridge page brought joy to our hearts as we looked forward to reading them every night.

Joan would later write these wonderful words to me, "In Yiddish there is a wonderful word, 'beshert' which means *meant to be.* It is often used in the sense of a romantic involvement, however most of us use it to mean all these connections. Isaac and your family were meant to come into my life." I'm a better parent because of the random acts of kindness by a stranger who till this day I've never met in person. Joan and her husband Joel never had children. Much like Dacia and I in our early years, when we contemplated loving someone else's child - when the gift of parenthood looked to pass us over. Reflecting on what Joan did for our family is a testament to the heart of what raising children should be for all parents – unconditional love. Joan met us at our time of need and earned a special place in our hearts.

One day soon, I promised Joan we would meet for dinner in Washington D.C. The reunion would not be between two strangers, but rather family getting together for the very first time.

Reverend Jon Greer
Youth Pastor
Sapulpa First Church of God
Sapulpa, Oklahoma

Growing up as a pastor's kid in Illinois, Jon Greer knew by the time he graduated high school he wanted to go into the ministry. Attending Mid-America Christian University in Oklahoma City, Jon earned his degree but finding a job as a pastor eluded him for a long time. Jon's first job upon graduation was serving as the sports marketing director at Mid America University. He later worked as a bank teller to provide for his young family. It was during this time Jon and his wife Katie had their first child. One lonely Saturday night, Jon decided to apply again for jobs in the ministry. He applied at five churches and received a call from the Sapulpa First Church of God. The church had been our home since 1998 and we were elated to have a young family man coming to serve as the youth pastor for our boys. Jon's third year in ministry at the Sapulpa church would be marred by a member of his youth group being diagnosed with cancer. Isaac Walsh had been diagnosed with medulloblastoma brain cancer. This would be a defining moment in Jon Greer's ministry.

Jon remarked nine years later, "Isaac's diagnosis was one of the most tragic things to happen in my life. There is no book on how to talk with a child facing death." Isaac and Jon developed a special friendship which transcended the bonds of a paternal caregiver. Isaac would share his worst fears with Pastor Jon. This special bond developed into a relationship in which Pastor Jon became the one person who could restore Isaac's will to live when the outcome looked bleak. Pastor Jon would reminisce years later, "I was scared, there were so many unknowns. There were times when I would come to the hospital and I had no idea what to expect." Jon had a two-year old son at the time of Isaac's cancer diagnosis. As a young father, Jon would often return home and find himself despondent as he contemplated what Isaac must be feeling. Fighting back tears as he looked into the eyes of his own child, Jon came to grips with how a loving God could allow a young child to suffer so much.

Isaac once told me Pastor Jon was the one person who had the biggest influence on his life throughout his treatment with cancer. In retrospect, Pastor Jon once told me, "Isaac knew all the textbook Bible story answers. I never told him I understood what he was going through. I allowed Isaac to talk about his worst fears." Isaac would text and talk with Jon almost every day during his time at St. Jude. The compassion and concern did not end when Isaac was discharged from the hospital. Rather, Jon realized cancer would alter Isaac's life forever. Pastor Jon forged a friendship with Isaac which has lasted to this day. In the latter years, Jon's counsel has been helping Isaac cope as a cancer survivor growing up in a normal world. Isaac had to adjust to a new normal the cancer treatment left behind.

As parents, my wife and I are eternally grateful for the healing hand of Pastor Jon. For months Jon was more than a Sunday fixture in our lives. He became the family member you call upon when your own instincts and plans become shattered by the unrelenting hardship imposed by cancer. We are a stronger family because of Pastor Jon. More so, our son is alive today because of Pastor Jon's compassion, and ability to motivate Isaac to never give up when the blanket of death attempted to smother his will to live. Pastor Jon is the epitome of what we expect from those in ministry today.

Helen Keller once said, "Walking with a friend in the dark is better than walking alone in the light." We are forever grateful to Pastor Jon for being a guiding light during our darkest days. His steadfast sympathy and kindred friendship forever changed our lives. As for Isaac, he appreciates Jon's compassion, and strives to be the example Jon set for him nine years ago.

Michelle Linn
FOX23 Morning News Anchor
Tulsa, Oklahoma

In 1996 a young St. Louis native landed a job at the ABC news affiliate station in Columbia, Missouri as a part-time reporter. Having graduated from William Woods University, this young professional would soon rise through the ranks of TV journalism. In a short time, she would quickly be promoted to a morning cut-in anchor during ABC's Good Morning America program. Her fourteen-year career at the Columbia station would take on many rolls including: news anchor, reporter, assignment desk editor, promotions manager and director of public relations. In 2010 Michelle Linn became a household name in Tulsa when she accepted a job as the morning co-host of FOX23 News. I met Michelle when our paths crossed after our return from St. Jude. In the spring of 2013, she was working on a segment for the Tulsa St. Jude Dream Home Giveaway, and we were called on to be a part of the story.

The ALSAC team at St. Jude put me in contact with Michelle as her station was local TV host of the Dream Home Giveaway. My first impression of Michelle later mirrored the story she produced – excellence. She was friendly and conveyed a sense of really wanting to understand Isaac's journey with cancer. Prior to meeting Michelle, I had previously done interviews at St. Jude regarding Isaac's cancer journey. A number of video clips had been put together regarding our time in Memphis. Years later, I would tell Michelle her narrative was the most heartfelt and sincere story ever done on Isaac's cancer diagnosis. I remember seeing the video for the first time. Tears filled my eyes as I relived the emotion of the day four powerful words changed our lives, "Your child has cancer." Unlike previous stories put together on Isaac's life, this one came from a reporter who understood the pain and suffering, only the parent of a cancer-stricken child could understand. It also was written by someone who had just returned from the very place which saved my child's life – Michelle had just returned from St. Jude.

Years later Michelle would recall the assignment - visiting St. Jude and producing a patient story. Originally, the task had been given to another anchor. However, the person resigned abruptly and went to another local station. Michelle had been given two weeks' notice to pack her bags and head east to Memphis. She told me prior to meeting the staff at St. Jude she was apprehensive and scared of what she might see. Children with cancer carried a life and death sentence which for most people was too heartbreaking and upsetting to be around. However, Michelle was awestruck by the ambiance of hope which is noticeable to all who visit St. Jude. She reiterated what I had come to know firsthand when she said, "St. Jude is not a sad place, I think it's because the people who work there are so exceptional. They have a gift for cultivating the most talented, compassionate, positive and caring employees. It was incredibly uplifting and a privilege to visit."

Michelle has visited the hospital every year since 2013 and produced stories on the patients and staff of St. Jude. I remembered her telling me seven years ago how it impacted her life in a powerful way. A person gains a deeper appreciation of the strength and courage it takes to overcome human suffering when seeing firsthand the work of St. Jude. For me, I admire the work of my dear friend Michelle and the commitment she makes to spread an awareness of pediatric cancer. Michelle once told me, "The stories of St. Jude families is the assignment I cherish the most." Anyone who knows Michelle cannot help but be drawn into her world of loving children, and be appreciative of her work on community projects. In a world where TV news is dominated by violence and crime, there are still some who view their most honorable and exemplary role is to be part of saving the life of a child.

Michelle, you are an extension of the brilliant, extraordinary, and kindhearted employees whom you have come to respect at St. Jude. You are part of the amazing St. Jude extended family, a family I joined in March of 2011 and my life has never been the same. The day I met you at the FOX23 news studio in Tulsa, Oklahoma *(in May 2013)* I was not only impressed by your passion for St. Jude, but for your amazing ability to convey the unbridled commitment I have for finding a cure for this devastating disease. It's a goal we both have, and one in which I'm forever grateful I got a chance to share with you.

Dr. Richard and Mrs. Janet Pitts
Godparents of Isaac and Caleb Walsh
Sapulpa, Oklahoma

Family and friends came from across the country to gather for our wedding on May 7, 1989 in Tulsa, Oklahoma. Dacia and I had come from two opposite worlds. She hailed from New Hampshire and I had spent the majority of my life growing up in north central Kansas. After graduation from Oral Roberts University, we both decided to look for teaching jobs in Oklahoma and make it our home. I remember in the early years having Thanksgiving dinner as a family of two. There were no brothers, sisters, aunts and uncles to share the special day as our nearest relatives were nearly four hundred miles away. I felt a subdued delight to be off work but yearned for the interaction of family during the holidays. For me, the day I walked into the dental office of Dr. Richard Pitts to be seen for an aching tooth, my yearning to have family close would never be the same.

I remember this first day I met him, he was outgoing and quite funny. His jovial and fun-loving personality comforted me during a stressful time. More so, his unique ability to empathize and explain in down to earth terms my dental condition led me to trust his judgement. Soon thereafter, I met Dr. Pitts again at a church function. Dacia and I were new members just getting to know those in the congregation. It was during this time, I got to know his outgoing and kindhearted wife Janet. Realizing we had no family in Oklahoma, they began inviting us to their large family gatherings during the holiday season. At first, I remember showing up as a stranger and hoping my intrusion would not be noticeable to those around me. However, in a short amount of time, I became part of this wonderful group of people. They would share in our joys when our kids were born and later grieve with us when Isaac was diagnosed with cancer.

Isaac spent his final day at the Pitts' home before being diagnosed with cancer. He was home from school and too fragile to be left alone. Despite having gone to numerous doctors and the emergency room only three days prior, our search for answers had yielded no results. In an effort to sooth his aching muscles, Isaac got into a hot tub. Janet would later reminisce Isaac was so weak, she had to go get her husband from the adjoining dental office to get him out. Richard's words nine years later would send chills down my spine as he said, "As I lifted him out of the tub, I looked into his eyes and it scared me. Isaac stared at me and I definitely knew something was wrong." Dr. Pitts would later call me at school during parent-teacher conferences and relay his concerns. It was upon his urging, I called our family pediatrician and told her, "If something is not done tonight, I doubt Isaac will be with us tomorrow. He is so frail and will not eat. He cannot walk nor is he able to get up from a seated position." Her words next would ring hollow as if they were repeated today, "Stay with Isaac and don't go anywhere. I'm going to call the children's hospital and have him admitted today." A few hours later, Isaac was admitted to St. Francis Children's Hospital in Tulsa, Oklahoma on March 8, 2011. Janet would recall the day she heard the report of Isaac's cancer diagnosis. She said, "The news took me to my knees. I was in tears." Despite no formal ancestral family connection, Isaac had become one of their own. Janet and Richard sacrificially made daily trips to the hospital in an effort to help us meet Isaac's needs. Approaching soon thereafter would be our trip to St. Jude, after joining a clinical trial in Memphis, Tennessee. Although Isaac was at the forefront of our concern, our thoughts soon became consumed by what we would do with our younger son Caleb.

I remember telling Dacia this long-extended absence required the help of family. There was no doubt we would need the help of Janet and Richard Pitts during our extended time away. Caleb would stay with his godparents for the next nine months. Having no children in their home at the time, Caleb brought back reminders of a having a young nine-year old elementary child. Richard remarked, "It was enjoyable having him here because none of our kids were into sports. I've never watched someone so good at soccer, he had to be pulled from the game after scoring so many goals." Janet and Richard would fulfill the role of parents as they went with Caleb to open house at school. Janet remarked, "We walked in with him and were by far the oldest ones in the room. We explained to the teacher we were Caleb's godparents. She took the time to explain to us how to complete the homework." They watched every soccer game and went on to see him run in his cross country meets. Janet and Richard began to take on the role of raising a child who viewed them as his parents. Janet would recall Caleb wanting to dress like her husband. Having remarked, "I remember Caleb asking for a peach colored dress shirt and navy-blue blazer just like Richard was wearing Sunday at church. He wanted to dress just like him." Janet would go out and buy the identical clothes for Caleb. In a surreal way, I can only think it brought a calm peace to Caleb's heart knowing he was living with two loving family members who cared for his every need.

Approximately six weeks after we arrived, Janet and Richard brought Caleb to Memphis for a visit. Janet's reaction after setting foot on the beautiful campus of St. Jude became more pronounced when she met with some of the medical staff. Janet said it best when she relayed, "The treatment alone combined with their expertise and care gave me hope Isaac would survive." Richard would remark, "It impressed me this was an international renowned hospital. I remember going into the St. Jude Chili's Care Center and realizing large corporations sponsor the work going on here."

Caleb would enjoy his frequent visits to Memphis, and we would trade off solo visits coming home. Each time we would stay with the Pitts family as our house had been "winterized," as if it were a vacation home. Richard would recall one of life's most difficult conversations when Caleb asked him if his older brother was going to die. Allowing Caleb to express his worst fears, Richard found this question difficult to answer. Caleb was old enough to understand cancer carries a penalty of death but yet viewed it only through a child's innocent eyes. Richard could only assure him Isaac was in the best place in the world and every effort was being made to save his life. Further, Caleb began to process the thought of losing his older brother by giving blanket answers to numerous questions thrown his way by saying, "Isaac is fine." At a young age, Caleb began to process the world through a hardened view of his brother's battle against cancer. However, he found a showering love and compassion by the Pitts family as if he were one of their very own.

Years later Caleb would remark, "It was like living at your grandparent's house and being a super spoiled grandkid." Notwithstanding, the lasting influence of Janet and Richard on Caleb's life would not end when we returned home from St. Jude. Caleb continues to frequent their home and even maintains a set of bathing suits in a dresser drawer in his old room. He uses them by going over to go swim in their pool. Just as a loving parent would offer advice and counsel to one of their children after leaving home, they still get questions from Caleb regarding his career, cars, girls and family. The impact of the Pitts family would not be on Caleb alone. During the two years Isaac spent in Memphis, he called every week as a dutiful son would his parents, when living so far away.

As for me, I am reminded of Dr. Pitts' phone call on March 8, 2011 which alerted us to a dangerous life-threatening situation. In retrospect, his insistence we seek medical care saved Isaac's life even before cancer treatments began. More so, Janet and Richard were more than a ceremonial family member who stands as godparents at a child's baptism, they were the life raft placed in our lives when all hope was lost. Our family would not have survived without the steadfast devotion, compassion and dedication of these two wonderful people who came into our world long before we had children. They were with us on the day Isaac was born and welcomed us home after we returned from St. Jude. We are continually blessed by their friendship and consider them family. Although, the miracle of Isaac returning home was seen by many as an answer to our prayers, noted British author and theologian C.S. Lewis put it best when he wrote...

"Miracles are a retelling in small letters of the very same story which is written across the whole world in letters too large for some of us to see."

Dr. Richard and Janet Pitts were the second part of the miracle which occurred in our lives. Through their tireless and unselfish efforts, we remained a strong family battered by the carnage of cancer but with two wonderful children who view it now as a distant painful memory. Forever family!

Earl and Sandy Blevins
Oklahoma Make a Wish Foundation

As lifelong Oklahomans, Earl and Sandy Blevins met during high school but did not come together as a family until thirty years later. When Sandy met her husband Earl later in adulthood, he was a dedicated Tulsa firefighter who was also a Make a Wish volunteer. Sandy would recall the time she went with her husband eleven years ago to interview a child for their "wish." After the interview, Sandy knew this was an organization she wanted to volunteer with on a regular basis. Almost like a parent who can name off the milestones in their child's life, Earl and Sandy can about their "wish," kids. Sandy has been involved in fundraising and has granted wishes for two hundred children. Earl lags behind at fifty-six, but reminds everyone up until six weeks ago he was working full time. He retired on June 12, 2020. Fighting a misconception the Make a Wish Foundation is only for kids with a terminal illness is a battle Sandy faces almost every day. Our family, was introduced to the Oklahoma Make a Wish Foundation after Isaac's brain surgery in Tulsa. Due to the critical nature of Isaac's surgery, he became a candidate for the program and was granted a wish. We would meet the coordinators for Isaac's "wish," while undergoing treatment at St. Jude.

Earl and Sandy Blevins had made their way to Memphis, but had never set foot on the beautiful grounds of St. Jude Children's Research Hospital. I suggested they take a guided tour and meet some of the exceptional staff. Sandy was overwhelmed by the magnificence of St. Jude. She would later say, "I was flabbergasted, it's like a whole new city." Earl recalls seeing a ying-yang symbol made up of words prominently placed in the patient care lobby. "Immediately, the words Make a Wish *(swirled within the symbol)* stood out to me," he said. Both Earl and Sandy would leave St. Jude with a sense of awe and astonishment at the work of such a wonderful dedicated group of professionals. More so, they met firsthand a child who was being treated there and wanted to do more. Earl went back to the Tulsa Fire Department and changed his payroll deduction to become a Partner in Hope for St. Jude. As for Isaac, he made his wish known – he wanted to go to Disney World in Orlando, Florida.

The plane was packed with children, all of whom were headed for Orlando. I could tell from the chatter around me, Disney was the destination of choice. We intentionally chose to take our trip in mid-December apart from the summer crowds and to avoid the heat of August. It had been almost an entire year since we returned home which gave Isaac time to heal and gain his strength. As we landed, a gentleman greeted us and brought us to a rental care agency. Since the bill had been paid in full, he loaded our bags into the car. We followed him to a Make a Wish retreat called *"Give Kids the World."*

The village is essentially a city in itself with apartments, cafeteria, arcade, bicycle path and park. The resort for Make a Wish children was started by Henri Landwirth who was known for his hotel businesses in Orlando. Henri was raised in a Jewish family in Antwerp, Belgium. During the outbreak of WWII, his family was captured and sent to the Nazi concentration camps. Separated from his parents, he spent six of his teenage years in Auschwitz and Mauthausen prisons. His parents would not survive the perils of mistreatment and torture. However, he and his twin sister Margot would endure the brutal persecution, only to be set free to rebuild their battered lives. Henri immigrated to America and joined the US Army in 1949. After serving as a soldier during the Korean War, he went to school on the GI bill and got a degree in hotel management. Soon thereafter, Mr. Landwirth became a prominent hotel and real estate mogul in the city of Orlando,

Florida. In the 1980's Henri began offering free hotel rooms to critically ill children visiting Disney with the Make a Wish Foundation. However, when a child died before travel arrangements could be made, Henri made a vow by writing, *"No child shall ever be failed again."* Today, the resort comprises 168 villas on 79 acres and is staffed by volunteers from all around the world. As we arrived on a warm December day, I remember the boys saying, "There is an arcade and it doesn't take coins – it's all free."

Prior to our trip, we had filled out a long questionnaire in regard to Isaac's health and special needs. Located within the village are medical doctors and nurses which volunteer their time to give kids the experience of a lifetime. Many children who come are critically ill and require a doctor's supervision. Others like Isaac are weak but proud to be living their dream. Further, the trip is for the entire family and not just the child who has suffered a life-threatening illness. Caleb remarked about the experience, "It was super sweet as with our *Make a Wish* badge we walked up the exits and got on the rides. We rode every ride in the park before lunch." Along with the special privileges on the Disney rides were passes to nearby Universal Studios, Harry Potter World and SeaWorld Park. In all, the entire trip lasted five days.

As we headed home, I could only think of Earl and Sandy Blevins who spearheaded the effort to give Isaac his "wish." Through their efforts more than $7,000 had been raised to make his dream come true. Earl and Sandy promised they would give him the world. It was a world in which every child is viewed as a precious gift of life. Judgement and ridicule do not exist. A blanket of love and compassion covers the scars of those who suffer from one of the undeserved tragedies of childhood. Prominently displayed at the Give Kids the World Resort, is a favorite quote of its founder Henri Landwirth:

"We make a living by what we get, we make a life by what we give." – Winston Churchill

I will always look back on this trip with fond memories. As a family, we are truly appreciative of the kindness of those who made it possible. More so by the commitment of two special people who give daily of themselves expecting nothing in return. Their dedication to grant the wish of a critically ill child is a standard we should all strive to live by.

Nicole Doyle
Senior Season Ticket Account Manager
NBA Oklahoma City Thunder

Growing up as the oldest of six children in Muskogee, *(Oklahoma)* Nicole Doyle took on the role of a big sister who helped raise her two younger sisters. Nicole would reminisce about the long hours her parents spent at their medical equipment supply business and the impact it had on the family. "My momma had me scrubbing the floors by the time I was in third grade. I washed my own clothes and took care of my younger sisters, one of whom was only a year old. She instilled in me a sense of independence which enabled me to confidently care for myself." Nicole would become the high school student who her younger sisters looked to in times of need. She took on the role of a loving parent who unselfishly gave of herself, to the benefit of those less fortunate. After graduation from Oklahoma State University, Nicole completed an event coordinator internship at the Ford Models firm in New York City. However, Nicole yearned to be closer to home and moved back to Oklahoma in 2011. It was the same year Isaac was diagnosed with cancer. I met this wonderful young woman when she had just been hired by the Oklahoma City Thunder as the marketing, programs and promotions coordinator.

The Oklahoma City Thunder played a pivotal role in Isaac's journey with cancer. He was their biggest fan and followed every game during our time in Memphis. Isaac wore his OKC Thunder jersey daily through the halls of St. Jude. Many of the doctors and nurses who were NBA fans found an avid follower who knew all the teams, stats and outlook for the playoffs. Isaac regularly discussed the OKC Thunder with St. Jude ALSAC CEO Rick Shadyac who was an enthusiastic fan of the NBA Memphis Grizzlies. Isaac would soon learn someone with the Oklahoma City Thunder had sought him out and wanted to connect with him.

Looking back, neither Nicole nor myself could pinpoint the day our paths crossed. My impression of the Thunder organization, through my interactions with Nicole, was this is first class. The people who worked for the team made a strong commitment to serve others and reach out to their community. Nicole would say it best when speaking of the very man who leads this outstanding organization when she said, "He is someone who I will become emotional when speaking about. He has the utmost integrity and the biggest heart in the world. I simply cannot say enough good things about our owner Clay Bennett." Mr. Bennett's influence became embedded in Nicole when she said, "I would like to believe it's in all of us, that when we see someone struggling, especially a child, our first innate reaction is to want to help and to let them know, if I can't make it better, I will sit here with you to get you through it." We would not meet Nicole until after we returned home from St. Jude. However, her kindness and generosity were felt during our stay in Memphis.

I remember telling Isaac someone with the Thunder named Nicole Doyle had reached out to me. In her email, she expressed sympathy for Isaac who at the time was undergoing brain cancer treatments at St. Jude. Further, she wanted our St. Jude mailing address as she wanted to send him something. Patiently Isaac waited and each day would ask if he received anything in the mail from Nicole Doyle. It finally came, waiting at the reception desk was a huge box addressed to Isaac Walsh from the Oklahoma City Thunder. I had no idea what Nicole had sent but decided to have my camera ready to capture his expression. My chin dropped to my knees when Isaac pulled from the box an autographed pair of OKC Thunder Forward Kevin Durant game shoes. Also, included was a team banner, schedule poster, Thunder jersey and a get-well card. Nicole spoke from the heart when she said, "I couldn't be more excited to have been given the opportunity to place those little milestones in his life. I think it's important when someone is struggling to sprinkler little things on their calendar for them to look forward to." As our time in Memphis was nearing the end, Nicole asked when we would be coming home. She wanted to meet us and send us first-class to a Thunder basketball game.

Walking into the Thunder corporate offices in downtown Oklahoma City, I was awestruck by the OKC Thunder gear displayed throughout the office. We were here to meet Nicole and attend a game. Nicole would later recall the encounter by saying, "I was nervous to meet him, *(Isaac)* it was emotional knowing what your family had been through." My first impression of Nicole was her beautiful beaming smile and outgoing personality which immediately put a stranger at ease. I was drawn to how dedicated she was to the Thunder organization, she was the star behind the scenes. Nicole brought us to the arena and showed us our suite, complete with food and drinks while we enjoyed the game. Because we got to the arena early, the boys got to meet with some of the players on the team, and return home with lots of autographs. Not to be outdone, a group of cheerleaders and even the team mascot *"Rumble,"* made a visit to our suite. It was a picture-perfect welcome home party, compliments of the NBA Oklahoma City Thunder – all arranged by Nicole Doyle.

The home arena of the Oklahoma City Thunder fills with thousands of fans for every home game, as all the contests are sellouts. The roaring crowd will cheer for their favorite players and shower them with praise. As for me, I think of a young twenty-six year-old recent college graduate who made the dreams of a cancer-stricken child come true. She was humble and wanted no attention. Her game stats were the compassion she bestowed on those less fortunate than her. Nicole once told me, "You get blessed, when they come into your life." Most importantly, Nicole brought a championship trophy to the feet of Isaac Walsh. She represents the best in sports today. Forever grateful!

Brian Davis
Fox Sports TV Play by Play Voice *(Retired)*
NBA Oklahoma City Thunder

His career would span four decades in professional and collegiate sports broadcasting. Tattooed on his resume are stints announcing games with virtually every American professional sports league including the National Football League, National Hockey League, National Basketball Association and Professional Soccer League. Colleges from coast to coast would see him sit courtside or in a press box to announce their games. The last stop in his storied career would be the Fox Sports play by play TV announcer with the Oklahoma City Thunder. It was during this time and while in Memphis, Tennessee - we met Mr. Brian Davis.

It was the NBA playoffs and the visiting Oklahoma City Thunder were in town to take on the Memphis Grizzlies at the downtown FedEx Forum. Prior to the start of the game, I went to the floor to find someone associated with the team in an attempt to bring the world of the NBA to my ailing son. In some ways, when I introduced myself to the familiar OKC Thunder TV personality, I didn't think anything would become of my encounter. Years later, Brian would reminisce by saying, "The night you came and introduced yourself to me in Memphis, the door opened. It was up to me to walk through it." On the other side of the door was the realm of St. Jude. It was a place Brian had seen at a distance but never felt compelled to explore the miracles which occurred there. Brian continued by saying, "Night to night you rarely find yourself placed in a special situation. It was the chance for me to be there for someone in a very minor way. It was the chance for me to walk the walk, I've always told myself I would." Brian's brief meeting with Isaac at the game would be the start of enduring friendship. Three days later Brian called and wanted to visit St. Jude.

Arriving at the campus of St. Jude, Brian gave his ID to the guard stationed at the gate. I had given his name to security and told them he would be coming for a family visit. Staring at the image of a praying child on the side of the building and seeing kids pulled in wagons, Brian realized he had arrived at a place reserved for families battling one of life's unforeseen tragedies – pediatric cancer. He recalled his emotions ten years later by saying, "For me, when I got a chance to walk through those gates, I felt like I was on hallowed ground. I knew enough about St. Jude to realize they are trying to make the lives of families and our world a better place." As he made his way to the hospital lobby, Isaac was there in a wheelchair eagerly waiting. For the first time since our journey with cancer began, the world of professional sports had come into our lives. Brian would recall the event by saying "Isaac faced this entire ordeal with equanimity. Every time I was around him there was a sense of serenity, his ability to face such a tough situation at such a young age is rare. It didn't break my heart rather it penetrated it." Brian marveled at the support Isaac received from his family. His heart went out to our younger son Caleb, who would have sacrificed so much for Isaac to receive the undivided attention he needed to survive. Cancer treatments would be a series of highs and lows for Isaac, and for his younger brother Caleb. Cancer carried a grave uncertainty of its outcome. This became evident to Brian when I reached out to him on September 30, 2011.

Brian recalled the day he received an email from me regarding a dire situation in which Isaac was admitted to the hospital and urgently needed brain surgery. The operation was placed on hold due to a bloodborne staph infection. A race against time ensued as without surgery, Isaac would pass away in a matter of only a few days. At the time, the NBA players were on strike and Brian was in Tampa to broadcast the NCAA Alabama vs. Florida football game. Normally the night before the event was a time to catch up with old friends whom he had known in the sports business. However, the weight of Isaac surrendering to the ills of cancer would leave him despondent and questioning the fragility of a young life. Carefully composing a return email, Brian remembered losing his best friend to colon cancer eleven years prior. The loss of his best friend prepared Brian to pen some difficult words. His response was not to give false hope at a time of expected loss. Rather, it sought to give perspective as I began to look at putting together my life after a bruising battle with childhood cancer. Brian agonized over his words, as he would later say, "I can't tell you how many hours I sat in my hotel room on Friday night composing an email back to you. I had no idea on how you would receive it." A section taken from Brian's email is noted below...

I do believe mere mortals can only take the fight so far. Beyond a certain point, illnesses of great magnitude whether on its own, or through complications which develop will take its course no matter how heroic the intervention. This is one of the issues I gather you're struggling with right now: What's fair to Isaac? How much to put him through? How much you can stand as you try to make decisions that hold such far-reaching and long-lasting implications, not only for Isaac but for your entire family? I believe Isaac will tell you how much he can tolerate. If the day comes that he's had enough, he'll let you know. If it comes to that, I also know this: He will take God's hand knowing how much you love him. How much you will always love him and how hard you tried to get him through this. If that day comes, you will be forever richer for his presence in your lives - in the good times and the bad.

Brian Davis
September 30, 2011 @ 10:52 PM

Brian's counsel would be a defining moment in my journey with Isaac's cancer. The next day I went to the graveside of Danny Thomas near the St. Jude Pavilion. The beautiful garden had become a place of meditation and solitude for me in times of trouble. I carefully reread Brian's email and found healing in his words. Isaac would let us know when he had enough. It would be his decision when he no longer wanted to keep fighting. In some respects, I let my fear of losing Isaac be replaced with an unrestrained peace which came after realizing it would be up to Isaac when he wanted to let go. The remaining three months of our time in Memphis would be the most difficult of the entire clinical trial. Recognizing only Isaac could fortify his will to survive, I saw my role as a loving parent who would provide him with the level of comfort he needed to make his own decisions on how far he wanted to take his fight. In the end, I could not force Isaac to get well nor change his attitude towards battling the disease.

Over the years, we would see Brian at every Thunder ballgame we attended. He was kind and generous making every effort to see us. Brian also made several appearances at fundraising events for St. Jude by agreeing to speak at the Tulsa area "Walk to End Cancer," rally held annually each September. As I contemplate what Brian's friendship has meant to me over the years, I came across a proverb which speaks to the heart of a man who walked through an "*open door*" when he left the floor of the Memphis FedEx Forum, and climbed the arena steps to meet a cancer stricken child.

Past the seeker as he prayed came the crippled and the beggar and the beaten. And seeing them, he cried. "Great God how is it that a loving creator can see such things and yet do nothing about them." God said, "I did do something. I made you." – Author unknown.

I'm a better person because of my relationship with Brian Davis. Forever friends and eternally grateful. – Tom Walsh

About the Author

T om Walsh grew up in north central Kansas in a small
farming community named Concordia. Calling the wheat
fields of Kansas his boyhood home, Tom was the oldest of
seven boys and one year younger than his sister Margie. At age
fifteen, Tom's parents moved their large family of eight kids to
Denver, Colorado in search of more opportunities for their
children. Upon graduation from high school, Tom attended
college in Tulsa, Oklahoma where he met his wife Dacia.
Deciding to plant their roots in the western suburbs of Tulsa,
Tom began his career teaching Spanish to junior high school
age students. It would be only six years later when he made the
transition to elementary school principal where he would spend
the remainder of his thirty-year career.

Tom retired after three decades in public education in the
year 2020. It was also the time our country was thrust into the
COVID-19 pandemic. Although his immediate retirement
plans were delayed, Tom began the process of writing his
oldest son Isaac's health story in an effort to spread an
awareness of pediatric cancer.

Currently, Tom frequently volunteers at El Shalom
Children's Orphanage and Brenner School in Santiago
Texacuangos, El Salvador. Relishing the opportunity to return
to the classroom, Tom reconnects with his past by being a
volunteer teacher to those less fortunate than him. He plans
twice annual trips to see the orphan children who have referred
to him as their "padrino." *(Spanish for godfather)*

Tom is an accomplished speaker who has spoken at
numerous fundraising events including the St. Jude Executive
Summit in New York City and the St. Jude Board of Directors
Meeting. During his time at St. Jude, he gave numerous

interviews to various media outlets and allowed his son's story to be used in marketing materials for fundraising purposes. In addition, Tom has spoken at several education conferences during his long tenure as a school leader.

Currently, Tom and his wife Dacia reside in Sapulpa, Oklahoma. Dacia having retired from public education in 2019, now works as a relationship banker at a local bank.

Tom is currently pursuing his dream to bring hope to the brokenhearted and healing to those whose lives have been upended by the permanent scars of pediatric cancer. For Tom, there is no greater honor than saving the life of a child. In a small way, Tom hopes by sharing his family's struggle it will further the research to find a cure for this horrible disease.

To get in touch with Tom, read his blog, see the gallery of pictures or follow his future writing endeavors visit:
www.thomasmwalsh.com

CPSIA information can be obtained
at www.ICGtesting.com
Printed in the USA
LVHW050328220621
690796LV00001BA/1